Trauma Stewardship

An Everyday Guide to Caring for Self While Caring for Others

Laura van Dernoot Lipsky
Connie Burk

EasyRead Large

Copyright Page from the Original Book

Trauma Stewardship

Copyright © 2009 by Laura van Dernoot Lipsky

All rights reserved. No part of this publication may be reproduced, distributed, or transmitted in any form or by any means, including photocopying, recording, or other electronic or mechanical methods, without the prior written permission of the publisher, except in the case of brief quotations embodied in critical reviews and certain other noncommercial uses permitted by copyright law. For permission requests, write to the publisher, addressed "Attention: Permissions Coordinator," at the address below.

Berrett-Koehler Publishers, Inc.
235 Montgomery Street, Suite 650
San Francisco, California 94104-2916
Tel: (415) 288-0260, Fax: (415) 362-2512
www.bkconnection.com

Ordering information for print editions

Quantity sales. Special discounts are available on quantity purchases by corporations, associations, and others. For details, contact the "Special Sales Department" at the Berrett-Koehler address above.

Individual sales. Berrett-Koehler publications are available through most bookstores. They can also be ordered directly from Berrett-Koehler: Tel: (800) 929-2929; Fax: (802) 864-7626; www.bkconnection.com

Orders for college textbook/course adoption use. Please contact Berrett-Koehler: Tel: (800) 929-2929; Fax: (802) 864-7626.

Orders by U.S. trade bookstores and wholesalers. Please contact Ingram Publisher Services, Tel: (800) 509-4887; Fax: (800) 838-1149; E-mail: customer.service@ingrampublisherservices.com; or visit www.ingrampublisherservices.com/Ordering for details about electronic ordering.

Berrett-Koehler and the BK logo are registered trademarks of Berrett-Koehler Publishers, Inc.

First Edition
Paperback print edition ISBN 978-1-57675-944-8
PDF e-book ISBN 978-1-60509-263-8

2009-1

Cartoons appearing on pages 2, 7, 10, 13, 17, 20, 22, 29, 40, 47, 49, 59, 61, 65, 67, 69, 70, 79, 81, 84, 90 94, 96, 99, 101, 103, 104, 108, 110, 112, 120, 122, 131, 134, 149, 167, 173, 181, 183, 185, 196, 201, 209, 211, 223, 230, 244 are al copyrighted to The New Yorker Collection. Licensed by Cartoonbank.com. All Rights Reserved.

"The Dream Keeper" (appearing on the cover and page vii) from *The Collected Poems of Langston Hughes*, edited by Arnold Rampersad, copyright 1994 by The Estate of Langston Hughes, reprinted with the permission of Alfred A. Knopf, a division of Random House, Incorporated, and Harold Ober Associates Incorporated.

Editors: Stacy Carlson and Karen Cook. Book producer and Designer: Yuko Uchikawa. Copyeditor: Elissa Rabellino. Proofreader: Debra Gates. Indexer: Rachel Rice.
Illustrations appearing on inside front and back cover by Andrea Thomas ©2007. Cover painting: Gianni Monteleone ©2007. Cover design: Yuko Uchikawa.

TABLE OF CONTENTS

More Praise for Trauma Stewardship	ii
FOREWORD	x
ACKNOWLEDGMENTS	xvi
ABOUT THE COAUTHOR	xxiv
INTRODUCTION: On the Cliff of Awakening	xxvii
PART ONE: Understanding Trauma Stewardship	1
CHAPTER ONE: A New Vision for Our Collective Work	2
CHAPTER TWO: The Three Levels of Trauma Stewardship	19
PART TWO: Mapping Your Response to Trauma Exposure	61
CHAPTER THREE: What Is Trauma Exposure Response?	62
CHAPTER FOUR: The 16 Warning Signs of Trauma Exposure Response	74
PART THREE: CREATING CHANGE FROM THE INSIDE OUT	211
CHAPTER FIVE: New Ways to Navigate	211
CHAPTER SIX: Coming into the Present Moment	241
PART FOUR: FINDING YOUR WAY TO TRAUMA STEWARDSHIP	267
CHAPTER SEVEN: Following the Five Directions	267
CHAPTER EIGHT: NORTH • Creating Space for Inquiry	274
CHAPTER NINE: EAST • Choosing Our Focus	325
CHAPTER TEN: SOUTH • Building Compassion and Community	350
CHAPTER ELEVEN: WEST • Finding Balance	400
CHAPTER TWELVE: THE FIFTH DIRECTION • A Daily Practice of Centering Ourselves	439
CONCLUSION: Closing Intention	475
NOTES	480
SELECTED BIBLIOGRAPHY	499

ABOUT THE AUTHOR	506
ABOUT BERRETT-KOEHLER PUBLISHERS	511
BE CONNECTED	514
THE FIVE DIRECTIONS	516
Index	517

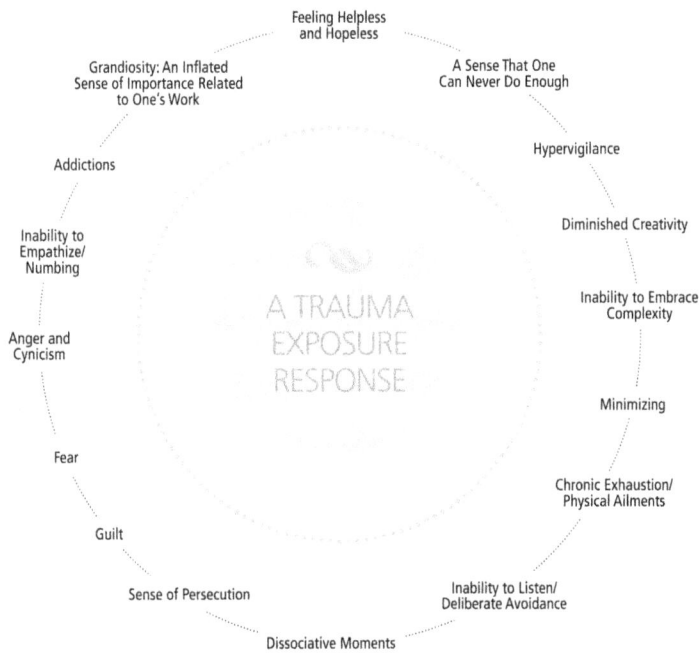

Figure A

More Praise for Trauma Stewardship

"Reading this book is like looking into a mirror. We will see ourselves much more clearly, will understand ourselves much better and will come up with better ways of being It and doing It. Compassion, yes, Compassion is Happiness itself. Enjoy."
—THICH NHAT HANH, Zen Master and peace activist

"Anyone who works with traumatized people can be caught in the grip of anxiety, irritability, or overwhelming sadness. By shutting out those feelings, you may sink into emotional numbness. You wish for wise words and a fresh perspective. You long for an understanding heart. You can find all that and more in Laura van Dernoot Lipsky's terrific book ... It will get you through hard times. It will help you feel better and work smarter. No trauma worker should be without it."

—GINNY NICARTHY, counselor, educator, and author of *Getting Free: You Can End Abuse and Take Back Your Life*

"*Trauma Stewardship* provides valuable advice for all those who toil for the betterment of society and the environment we share. Author Laura van Dernoot Lipsky's lifetime of caring and service has given her powerful insights into those who have similarly devoted their lives to the greater good. She reminds us all to embrace the joy of connecting with the people and planet that we cherish and serve."
—JOHN FLICKER, President and CEO, National Audubon Society

"Laura makes a superb case for 'trauma stewardship' as an approach that will benefit all of us in the service community who must deal with the struggles of our work with a hurting world. Her real-life stories hit home and clearly illustrate the ways that the traumatic situations we experience at work can carry into our personal view of our world. Laura helps us understand our own responses to trauma and

provides a path of renewal. Her book offers tools to bring us back to a place of balance where we can be more effective in our work, more present with our families, and more importantly, more at peace in our own soul."
 —MICHAEL L. TUGGY, MD, Director, Swedish Medical Center Family Medicine Residency Program; Medical Director, Swedish Family Medicine First Hill Clinic; and recipient of the Bronze Star from the US Army

"Laura van Dernoot Lipsky and *Trauma Stewardship* gave me language to describe what I was feeling after three trips to Iraq and subsequent work among US service members struggling to heal from war. *Trauma Stewardship* helped me acknowledge that my pain was not weakness to be suppressed or anesthetized but secondary trauma. But perhaps most important, *Trauma Stewardship* has shown me a path—not an easy one, to be sure, but a concrete one—toward a better and healthier life."
 —BRIAN PALMER, journalist

"Having been an attorney for only two years, I was both surprised and relieved to recognize many signs of secondary trauma in myself. Surprised because I had never been able to acknowledge the impact of my work as a public defender in such a way; relieved for the very same reason. I have come to rely on this book as a means to help me bear the weight of what can feel like inexorable human tragedy. It is *only* through the practices articulated and encouraged in *Trauma Stewardship* that my spirit remains intact. Each person I represent is better served for my having used this book. I recommend it to every public interest attorney and law student."
—ELIZABETH LATIMER, public defense attorney, Brooklyn Defender Services

"It is extremely easy, especially as caregivers, to overlook ourselves and our care. Laura takes us, the trauma stewards, on a journey of self-healing: her book's humor will make you laugh; its tools will help make us whole. She reminds us that the work we do as caregivers not only impacts our clients

but also deeply affects us. *Trauma Stewardship* provides us with methods to help us get in touch with habits and feelings that no longer serve us, our communities, or our work. A must-read for all those who understand that this work we do is sacred."
—KANIKA TAYLOR-MURPHY, community activist

"Laura is a weaver. She takes the harsh yet resilient fibers that are the stories of trauma survivors and workers, including her own, threads them together with common-sense advice, and creates a warm and soft blanket that comforts and protects. It is an important book because it reminds you to care for yourself as you care for others and then offers practical tools for doing so. I wish I'd had this book when I first began my work with women and children experiencing domestic violence!"
—GRETCHEN TEST, Program Associate for Child Welfare, Annie E. Casey Foundation

"In this groundbreaking guide to trauma stewardship, van Dernoot Lipsky shines new light on the care of the healers in the helping professions and provides a useful and loving guide to developing our ability to care for ourselves as much as we care for others. Anyone in the helping professions will benefit from the profound insights offered in this book."
—MIA EISENSTADT, consultant, activist, and anthropologist

For my ancestors and the sacred wilderness that surrounds me

The Dream Keeper
by Langston Hughes

Bring me all of your dreams,
You dreamers,
Bring me all of your
Heart melodies
That I may wrap them
In a blue cloud-cloth
Away from the too-rough fingers
Of the world.

FOREWORD

When my friend and colleague Laura van Dernoot first told me she was thinking of writing a book on secondary trauma, my first internal reaction went something like, "That is the last thing the world needs." She will no doubt remind me if my internal reaction was actually externalized in words. (You who are about to enjoy this book will get a glimpse into the tell-the-truth-with-loving-concern person that Laura is.)

Whether I said it out aloud or only in my own head, my concern was that in many pieces of literature, notions of vicarious trauma (a.k.a. empathic strain, compassion fatigue, secondary trauma, burnout) are being thrown around with little appreciation for what they mean or what taking them seriously would require of us. (The same is true for many other meaningful concepts, including evidence-based practice, cultural competence, and authenticity.) Poor practice, errors in practice, agency insensitivity to employees, rudeness among colleagues, tardiness, sloppiness, and other minor and major events taking place in practice today are excused as "secondary trauma." All kinds of work-related stress, emotional or behavioral responses to the demands of the workplace, and other work-related conditions are also fluffed off as "secondary trauma."

You will find in the pages that follow that Laura has a keen understanding of trauma and the responses to it. This is a book written by someone who has walked the path and knows firsthand what trauma brings and demands of those who walk that path. Her honesty, humor, and no-nonsense approach make these vital topics accessible to all of us. Even the most experienced trauma worker will find a refreshing perspective here. Her idea of trauma stewardship is a great gift to our field. It erodes the artificial line between sufferer and helper. It recognizes that trauma has impacts that can be named and managed. Trauma stewardship calls into question whether the means of exposure (direct or indirect, through relationships with those directly exposed) has any relevance to the impact of the trauma. Most of all, trauma stewardship calls on us to remember that it is a gift to be present when people deal with trauma; it reminds us of our responsibility to care and to nurture our capacity to help.

You will soon read Laura's claim that she brings no new knowledge to this calling. This is far from the truth. Not only is trauma stewardship a new formulation, but in ways that no other book or trainer has done, Laura links the key components of responding to trauma together in a way that is seamless and natural. One cannot go away from this book without understanding the relationship between oppression and trauma, the importance of purposeful action to protecting others and self, and the vital role that spirituality plays in protecting us from and managing trauma's impact on our own lives, as well as on the lives of our clients and friends. It interests me that Laura comes to this appreciation of the role of spirituality from walking the path, although increasingly this is also a finding from research on vicarious trauma.

Laura directs our attention to the impacts of trauma work on those who help and witness. Rather than pathologizing those of us who experience these reactions at one time or another, she helps us to understand our feelings and behavior as natural responses that flow from our humanity. In the same way that oils splatter on the painter's shirt or dirt gets under the gardener's nails, trauma work has an impact. As psychotherapists, we know that when the sources of anxiety go unrecognized, the anxiety cannot be managed. When that is the case, not only we but also our clients may suffer unnecessary distress. Laura gives us a range of possible emotions, ideas, and behaviors that can indicate that the work is taking a toll.

Perhaps the greatest gift this book gives us lies in the sections on finding compasses. Instead of producing a cookbook, Laura takes us along on her own journey. The Five Directions invite us, it seems to me, on a single direction that is inward so we can again go outward to the work. I haven't told Laura until now that when I first read this, I was angry. "Laura, for heaven's sake"—maybe the real words were a bit stronger—"tell me what to do!" Then I came to understand, as I took the deep breath she invites her reader to take, that the answer for her cannot be the answer for me. She gives us a compass, but each of us has to find the direction.

Those of you who are about to read this book are at the trailhead of a path that holds great promise for you, for your work, and for those whom you are privileged to work with. In an age when the same ideas get repeated until they lose any meaning, this is a book with fresh ideas. Unlike cookbooks or manuals that invite quick responses that have not been thought out, this book invites us on a journey. On that journey, we are invited to take a fresh look at why we do the work, and how our work must be contextualized in efforts to end oppression and privilege. We are reminded that the work has inevitable benefits and challenges, that we are stewards not just of those who allow us into their lives but of our own capacity to be helpful, and that a mindful and connected journey, both internally and externally, allows us to sustain the work.

We are in this work together, all of us. Our best hope is to understand that it is a long journey. We need to take care of ourselves and each other. Laura has given us a great compass and map to help us on our journey.

JON R. CONTE, PH.D.
Seattle, Washington

ACKNOWLEDGMENTS

There is no end to the people to whom I offer thanks for their much-needed help in writing this book. I am grateful to Aliyah and Mikaela, for teaching me what it truly means to have faith and for forgiving me each and every time I said, *"Solamente dos más minutos"*—a promise on which I could rarely deliver. To Joshua, who is my greatest role model, for reminding me what is truly important in life, and for helping me find my way back home. To Craig, who was the first to help me get back on my feet in life when I fell. To my father, who gifted me with an understanding of what it means to be grateful for my surroundings. To my mother, who gifted me with my passion and whose spirit kept me company throughout the process of writing. To Margarita Gutierrez, for being my sister and showing me what an open heart looks like. To Connie Burk and Jake Fawcett, whom we are proud to call our family and our friends, who inspire us with ceaseless generosity, and who are largely responsible for this book's emergence. To Caleb, who taught me what it means to be present. To Richard Appelbaum, for helping me connect with the rest of my life. To Jon Conte, whose willingness to sit with me and to bring true joy and great clarity has been unconditional and whose wisdom has allowed me to pursue this path. To Billie Lawson, who was a lifeline after many graveyard shifts, and whose humor has taught me so much. To Heather Andersen and Leslie Christian, for being deeply inspiring friends and beautiful mentors, and for their wonderfully generous financial support. To Michael Lipsky, whose tough love and belief in me helped form the foundation for my writing. To David Andrew, whose honesty and commitment to what could be helped the book truly come into its own. To Jerry Litner, who provided the wisdom that led me to a critical turning point, and to Suzanne Litner, for her care and practical support of the book. To Shayna Berkowitz and Phyllis Wiener, for their thoughtful donation to the book. To Charlie Browne, for inviting me to live in gratitude and start anew.

To Harry, Anna, Helen, Vance, Cindy, Deadria, Heather, Cheri, Polly, Warren, Vicky, Donna, and Jonathan, whose insights, honesty, and wisdom inspired my efforts to create a place that would be worthy of holding their stories. To Charles Newcomb, Sarah Bexell, Luo Lan, Jill Robinson, L.P., Kati Loeffler, Kirsten Stade, Victor Pantesco, Karen Lips, Chihchun, and Nancy Dammann, for helping me to realize my dream of connecting this work with their efforts to protect animals and ecosystems worldwide. To Zaid Hassan, whose friendship, encouragement, and feedback provided tremendous support. To Eli Kimaro, whose confidence and refusal to collude with my doubts allowed for critical forward motion. To Ginny NiCarthy, who has generated light and strength for me for two decades. To James and Linda Mooney, George Bertelstein, and Karena Goldfinger, for their love, for letting me sit at their feet, and for keeping the mirror dusted off. To Claire Guyu Johnson, for lighting the way inward. To Jack Kornfield, for his openness to collaborating with me, which has given me a gift I'll always cherish. To Thây, for creating a world I did not know was possible and for inviting me to walk along with him. To Jane Hansberry, Laurie Leitch, Elaine Miller-Karas, and Kathleen Tyrrell, for their warm welcome and invaluable sharing. To Felix, Hanna, Saskia, Tina, and Mark, for reminding me daily of what is truly possible. To Yanet Moo Chan, Laurence Opiniano, and Michelle Opiniano for critical communal parenting. To all who have provided feedback, critique, enthusiasm, introductions, and reminders that they care about this work, including Steve Tan, Robert Ruvkun, Mariette Newcomb, Ron Slye, Jacob Lipsky, Suzanne Goren, Stephanie Levine, Phyllis Barajas, Ingrid Dankmeyer, Claudia Carreño, Issraella Kleiman, Rivy Kletenik, Kym Anderson, Aislyn Colgan, Erin Healy, Holly Morris Bennet, Mia Eisenstadt, Shelly Shapiro, Julie Edsforth, Jay Katz, Abbey Semel, Russell Saunders, Jayasiddhi, Theresa LaLanne, Lisa Willis, Maia Olson, Lisa Fitzhugh, Sister Pine, Lavinia Browne, Sister Susan, Louise Ste. Marie, Joseph Rodríguez, Melissa Winter, Heather Higginbottom, Chris Lu, Laura

Amazzone, Garry Trudeau, Colin Kopes-Kerr, Adam Vogt, Eric Semel, Michele Matrisciani, Jon Bergevin, Marc Heusner, Jason Robertson, Jayna Gieber, Tom Kenney, Erin Galvin, Karyn Schwartz, Cynthia Garrett, Michael Tuggy, Kanika Taylor-Murphy, Grethen Test, Chelsea Sexton, Norm Stamper, John Flicker, David Olson, Benjamin Schonbrun, Tom Johnson, Robyn Nordstrom-Lane, Laura Simms, Dean Ericksen, Karen Maeda Allman, Data Reproductions, Megan Sukys, Jeremy Richards, Tim Taylor, Lisa DiMartino, Brian Palmer, Elizabeth Latimer, Jamie Willis, Christie Schmid, Tara Wolfe, Barbara Casey, Daniel Siegel, Brother Pháp Hưũ, Brother Phíp Trì, Debra Gates, Rachel Rice, Betsy Model, and independent bookstores around the United States. To Jay Katz, Toby Cox, Rachel VanDeMark, Ann Sonz Matranga, David Kerns, Janice Rutledge, Jenny Williams, and Donna Calame, whose investment in and dedication to our work, along with tremendous generosity, allowed us to go even deeper and aspire to even greater heights. To Rinku Sen, for her sincere support of our work, for her inspiring guidance, and for an invaluable introduction to Berrett-Koehler. To Johanna Vondeling and Jeevan Sivasubramaniam, for truly understanding our intention with this book and for welcoming us into their world with unparalleled faith, generosity, kindness, skill, and humor. For all those at Berrett-Koehler: I am eternally grateful for the opportunity to work with them and have one more chance to create this book. To Samantha Wipperman, for her endless belief in this work and her ever-present kindness. To Merrideth Miller and all the fabulous *New Yorker* cartoonists who have sustained my laughter over the years. To Jessica Stockton Bagnulo, for her spectacular attention to detail and a final read-through that gave us peace of mind. To Elissa Rabellino, for her willingness to go so above and beyond, and for the grace and talent with which she does her work. To Andrea Thomas, for her care in translating the concepts into wonderful visuals. To Britt Martin and Gianni Monteleone, for being such loving comrades and for blessing this work with their tremendous artistry.

To my profoundly talented editors Stacy Carlson and Karen Cook, whose endless generosity, kindness, commitment, and phenomenal editorial abilities breathed the necessary life and form into each and every sentence. This book could never have been anything close to what follows if not for their brilliance and exquisite vision.

To Yuko Uchikawa, whose loving friendship and steadfast confidence in this work has been a great blessing and a critical factor in this c book's evolution. Her intuition, wisdom, and marvelous artistic ability are what allow you to hold what you have in your hand.

And to all those valiant souls with whom I have had the privilege of working since I was 18 years old. I hope this book is worthy of all you have contributed to it, and I ask your forgiveness for any ways in which I was not capable of being as present as you deserved during our times together. I carry all of you in my heart and hope that the lessons I have learned and applied may allow others to be well served through the work of trauma stewardship. I feel humble in the presence of your spirits, and I am deeply honored to have your company on this path.

ABOUT THE COAUTHOR

Connie Burk is one of the primary reasons this book exists. Were it not for her vision, generosity, and faith in me, the text would still be floating around in my head. I am forever grateful to have had such an exquisite coauthor throughout the entire process. Connie urged me to turn my ideas about trauma stewardship into a book, and she refused to agree with me when I repeatedly said, "I am so not a writer!" She provided crucial perspective on the book as a whole and invited me to explore and reexplore my beliefs in a way that brought unprecedented depth to my work. Connie has a level of historical knowledge that was essential, and she role-modeled being patient as we tried to put our stream of thoughts into written words. She held the entirety of the process in a joyful embrace.

I met Connie years ago, when she first moved to Seattle. She had been recruited to be the executive director of the Northwest Network of Bisexual, Trans, Lesbian and Gay Survivors of

Abuse. Shortly after she arrived, I was asked to work with the organization as an advocate. Connie and I had our first meeting some days into my employment there. Sitting across from me, she asked what I would need to do my work well and how she could be of help. I told her that wherever I did direct service, I made sure to receive outside consultation twice a month to discuss the impact of the work on me, and that I'd need the Network to cover that. There was a memorably long pause. Eventually Connie said, "I had in mind something more in the shape of a muffin."

While obviously we did not start out on the same page about trauma stewardship, Connie is in large part responsible for anything you may glean from this book.

You can only go halfway into the darkest forest; then you're coming out the other side.

                              Chinese proverb

INTRODUCTION

On the Cliff of Awakening

"Are you sure all this trauma work hasn't gotten to you?" he asked.

We were visiting our relatives in the Caribbean. We had hiked to the top of some cliffs on a small island, and for a moment the entire family stood quietly together, marveling, looking out at the sea. It was an exquisite sight. There was turquoise water as far as you could see, a vast, cloudless sky, and air that felt incredible to breathe. As we reached the edge of the cliffs, my first thought was, "This is unbelievably beautiful." My second thought was, "I wonder how many people have killed themselves by jumping off these cliffs."

Assuming that everyone around me would be having exactly the same thought, I posed my question out loud. My stepfather-in-law turned to me slowly and asked his question with such sincerity that I finally understood: My work *had* gotten to me. I didn't even tell him the rest of what I was thinking:

"Where will the helicopter land? Where is the closest Level 1 trauma center? Can they transport from this island to a hospital? How long will that take? Does all of the Caribbean share a trauma center?" It was quite a list. I had always considered myself a self-aware person, but this was the first time I truly comprehended the degree to which my work had transformed the way that I engaged with the world.

That was in 1997. I had already spent more than a decade working, by choice, for social change. My jobs had brought me into intimate contact with people who were living close to or actually experiencing different types of acute trauma: homelessness, child abuse, domestic violence, substance abuse, community tragedies, natural disasters. As I continued on this path, my roles had grown and shifted. I had been an emergency room social worker, a community organizer, an immigrant and refugee advocate, an educator. I had been a front-line worker and a manager. I had worked days, evenings, and graveyard shifts. I had worked in my local community, elsewhere in the United States, and internationally.

Over time, there had been a number of people—friends, family, even clients—urging me to "take some time off," "think about some other work," or "stop taking it all so seriously." But I could not hear them. I was impassioned, perhaps to the point of selective blindness. I was blazing my own trail, and I believed that others just didn't get it. I was certain that this work was my calling, my life's mission. I was arrogant and self-righteous. I was convinced that I was just fine. (Figure B)

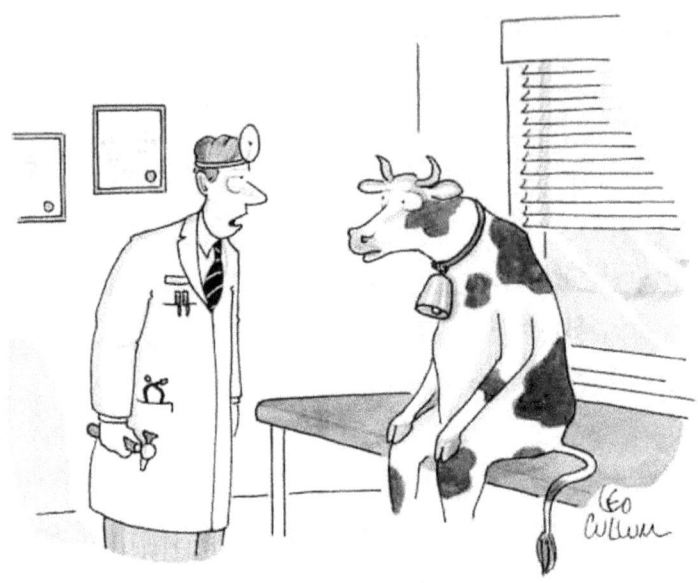

Figure B: "The ringing in your ears—I think I can help."

And so in that moment, on those cliffs, my sudden clarity about the work's toll on my life had a profound impact. Over the next days and weeks, I slowly began to make the connections. Not everyone stands on top of cliffs wondering how many people have jumped. Not everyone feels like crying when they see a room full of people with plastic lids on their to-go coffee containers. Not everyone is doing background checks on people they date, and pity is not everyone's first response when they receive a wedding invitation.

After so many years of hearing stories of abuse, death, tragic accidents, and unhappiness; of seeing photos of crime scenes, missing children, and deported loved ones; and of visiting the homes of those I was trying to help—in other words, of bearing witness to others' suffering—I finally came to understand that my exposure to other people's trauma had changed me on a fundamental level. There had been an osmosis: I had absorbed and accumulated trauma to the point that it had become part of me, and my view of the world had changed. I realized eventually that I had come into my work armed with a burning passion and a tremendous commitment, but few other internal resources. As you know, there is a time for fire, but what sustains the heat—for the long haul—is the coals. And coals I had none of. I did the work for a long time with very little ability to integrate my experiences emotionally, cognitively, spiritually, or physically.

Rather than staying in touch with the heart that was breaking, again and again, as a result of what I was witnessing, I had started building up walls. In my case, this meant becoming increasingly cocky. I had no access to the humility that we all need if we are to honestly engage our own internal process. Rather than acknowledge my own pain and helplessness in the face of things I could not control, I raged at the possible external causes. I sharpened my critique of systems and society. I became more dogmatic, opinionated, and intolerant of others' views than ever before. It never occurred to me that my anger might in part be functioning as a shield against what I was experiencing. I had no clue that I was warding off anguish, or that I was secretly terrified that I wouldn't be able to hold my life together if I lost my long-held conviction that all could be made well with the world if only we could do the right thing. Without my noticing it, this trail I was blazing had led me into a tangled wilderness. I was exhausted and thirsty, and no longer had the emotional or physical supplies I needed to continue.

    I could have ignored the realization that began on those cliffs. In the fields where I work, there is historically a widely held belief that if you're tough enough and cool enough and committed to your cause enough, you'll keep on keeping on, you'll suck it up: Self-care is for the weaker set. I had internalized this belief to a large degree, but once I realized that this way of dealing with trauma exposure was creating deep inroads in my life, I could not return to my former relationship with my work.

Instead, I began the long haul of making change. I knew that if I wanted to bring skill, insight, and energy to my work, my family, my community, and my own life, I had to alter my course. I had to learn new navigational skills. First, I needed to take responsibility for acknowledging the effects of trauma exposure within myself. Second, I had to learn how to make room for my own internal process—to create the space within to heal and to discover what I would need to continue with clarity on my chosen path. I had to find some way to bear witness to trauma without surrendering my ability to live fully. I needed a new framework of meaning—the concept that I would eventually come to call *trauma stewardship*.

Seung Sahn, the founder of the Kwan Um School of Zen, once said, "The Great Way is easy; all you have to do is let go of all your ideas, opinions, and preferences." Following his advice, I began to reconnect with myself. I learned how to be honest about how I was doing, moment by moment. I put myself at the feet of a great many teachers, medicine people, healers, brilliant minds, and loved ones. I asked for help. I began to reengage the wilderness around my home and to learn all the lessons I could from the endless intermingling of beauty and brutality that makes us so keenly feel the preciousness of life in the natural world. I began a daily practice that has allowed me to be present for my life and my work in a way that keeps me well and allows me to work with integrity and to the best of my ability.

Ultimately, I recognized that it was ego that had motivated me to keep on keeping on in my work long after I stopped being truly available to my clients or myself. Over the years, I gradually let go of that façade, and I reached a deep understanding of how our exposure to the suffering of others takes a toll on us personally and professionally. The depth, scope, and causes are different for everyone, but the fact that we are affected by the suffering of others and of our planet—that we have a *trauma exposure response*—is universal.

Trauma exposure response is only slowly coming to the fore as a larger social concern rather than simply an issue for isolated individuals. It was first recognized a decade ago in family members of Holocaust survivors and spouses of war veterans, but it has only recently attracted wide attention from researchers, who are working to assess its broader societal implications. To cite one example: According to a March 2007 *Newsweek* article, a U.S. Army internal advisory report on health care for troops in Iraq in 2006 indicated that 33 percent of behavioral-health personnel, 45 percent of primary-care specialists, and 27 percent of chaplains described feeling high or very high levels of "provider fatigue." The article concluded with this blunt appraisal: "Now homecoming vets have to deal with one more kind of collateral damage: traumatized caregivers."

In 2007, CNN.com published an article by Andree LeRoy, M.D., titled "Exhaustion, anger of caregiving get a name." It begins, "Do you take care of someone in your family with a chronic medical illness or dementia? Have you felt depression, anger or guilt? Has your health deteriorated since taking on the responsibility of caregiving? If your answer is yes to any one of these, you may be suffering from caregiver stress." The article reports a finding by the American Academy of Geriatric Psychiatrists that one out of every four families in the United States is caring for someone over the age of 50, with projections that this number will increase dramatically as the population in America ages. Another source for the article is Peter Vitaliano, a professor of geriatric psychiatry at the University of Washington and an expert on caregiving. He reports that many caregivers suffer from high blood pressure, diabetes, a compromised immune system, and other symptoms that can be linked to prolonged exposure to elevated levels of stress hormones. Unfortunately, many "don't seek help because they don't realize that they have a recognizable condition," the article says. In addition, Vitaliano explains, "caregivers are usually so immersed in their role that they neglect their own care." The article cites online conversations among caregivers who acknowledge that in such an emotional state, it's difficult to provide high-quality care to their loved ones.

While most research to date has concentrated on the effects of trauma exposure on those who watch humans suffer, we know that responding to trauma exposure is critical for those who bear witness to tragedies afflicting other species as well. Among these are veterinarians, animal rescue workers, biologists, and ecologists. We cannot ignore emerging information about the profound levels of trauma exposure among people in the front lines of the environmental movement—those fighting to stop the juggernaut of global warming and those who strive desperately, in the face of mounting losses, to ward off the extinction of countless species of plants and animals.

Pioneering researchers have given our experience of being affected by others' pain a number of names. In this book, we refer to "trauma exposure response." Charles Figley uses the terms "compassion fatigue" and "secondary traumatic stress disorder." Laurie Anne Pearlman, Karen W. Saakvitne, and I. L. McCann refer to the process as "vicarious traumatization." Jon Conte uses the words "empathic strain." Still others call it "secondary trauma."

Here, we include trauma exposure response under a larger rubric: *trauma stewardship.* As I see it, trauma stewardship refers to the entire conversation about how we come to do this work, how we are affected by it, and how we make sense of and learn from our experiences. In the dictionary, *stewardship* is defined as "the careful and responsible management of something entrusted to one's care." These days, the term is widely used in connection with conservation and natural-resource management. In the

January 2000 issue of the *Journal of Agricultural and Environmental Ethics,* Richard Worrell and Michael Appleby defined *stewardship* as taking care "in a way that takes full and balanced account of the interests of society, future generations, and other species, as well as of private needs, and accepts significant answerability to society."

When we talk about trauma in terms of stewardship, we remember that we are being entrusted with people's stories and their very lives, animals' well-being, and our planet's health. We understand that this is an incredible honor as well as a tremendous responsibility. We know that as stewards, we create a space for and honor others' hardship and suffering, and yet we do not assume their pain as our own. We care for others to the best of our ability without taking on their paths as our paths. We act with integrity toward our environment rather than being immobilized by the enormity of the current global climate crisis. We develop and maintain a long-term strategy that enables us to remain whole and helpful to others and our surroundings even amid great challenges. To participate in trauma stewardship is to always remember the privilege and sacredness of being called to help. It means maintaining our highest ethics, integrity, and responsibility every step of the way. In this book, I will attempt to provide readers with a meaningful guide to becoming a trauma steward.

The essayist E.B. White once wrote that the early American author, naturalist, and philosopher Henry Thoreau appeared to have been "torn by two powerful and opposing drives—the desire to enjoy the world, and the urge to set the world straight." This book is written for anyone who is doing work with an intention to make the world more sustainable and hopeful—all in all, a better place—and who, through this work, is exposed to the hardship, pain, crisis, trauma, or suffering of other living beings or the planet itself. It is for those who notice that they are not the same people they once were, or are being told by their families, friends, colleagues, or pets that something is different about them. (Figure C)

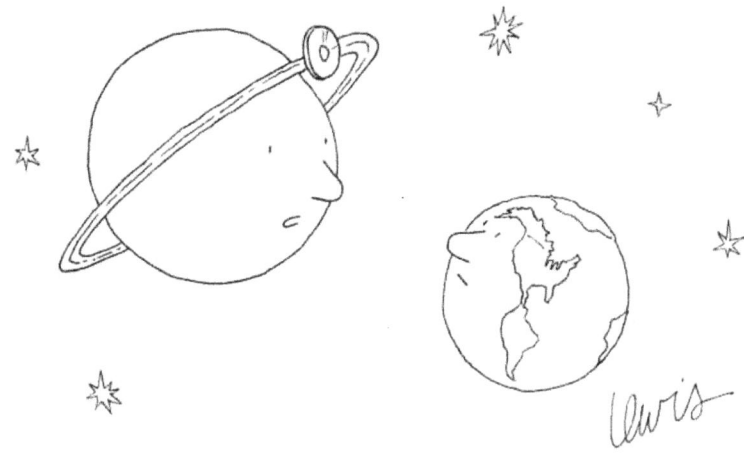

Figure C: "I'm afraid you have humans."

If even a few of the readers of this book can enhance their capacity for trauma stewardship, we can expect to see consequences, large and small, that will extend beyond us as individuals to affect our organizations, our movements, our communities, and ultimately society as a whole. In part 1, I talk more about what trauma stewardship is and how we can embark on our journey of change. Since the first step toward repair is always to understand what isn't working, I've devoted part 2 to mapping our trauma exposure response. Many readers may be startled by how intimately they already know the 16 warning signs I present in chapter 4.

Even if you haven't experienced these feelings or behaviors yourself, you are certain to know others who have.

How do we escape the constriction and suffering that often accompany trauma exposure response? In part 3, I provide some general tips, along with an in-depth exploration of the importance of coming into the present moment. In part 4, I offer the Five Directions, a guide that combines instructions for personal inquiry with practical advice that can greatly enhance our ability to care for ourselves, others, and the planet. I have included numerous brief exercises that you may choose to try as you develop your daily practice. Throughout the book, you will encounter profiles of inspiring people, perhaps much like you, who are deeply committed to the struggle to reconcile the hardships and joys of doing this work. As we illuminate the path of trauma stewardship, we will also shine light on the larger contexts in which we interact with suffering. We will delve deeply into how to carefully and responsibly manage what is being entrusted to us.

This book is a navigational tool for remembering that we have options at every step of our lives. We choose our own path. We can make a difference without suffering; we can do meaningful work in a way that works for us and for those we serve. We can enjoy the world *and* set it straight. We can leave a legacy that embodies our deepest wisdom and greatest gifts instead of one that is burdened with our struggles and despair.

As the author of this book, I don't believe that I am imparting new information. Rather, I'm offering reminders of lore that people from different walks of life, cultural traditions, and spiritual practices have known for millennia. There is a Native American teaching that babies come into the world knowing all they will need for their entire lifetimes—but the challenges of living in our strained, confusing world make them forget their innate wisdom. They spend their lives trying to remember what they once knew. (Some say this is the reason why the elderly and very young children so often have a magical connection: One is on the cusp of going where the other just came from.) This book aims to guide you, the reader, in finding a way home to yourself. All of the wisdom you are about to encounter is known to you already. This text is simply a way to help you remember.

PART ONE

Understanding Trauma Stewardship

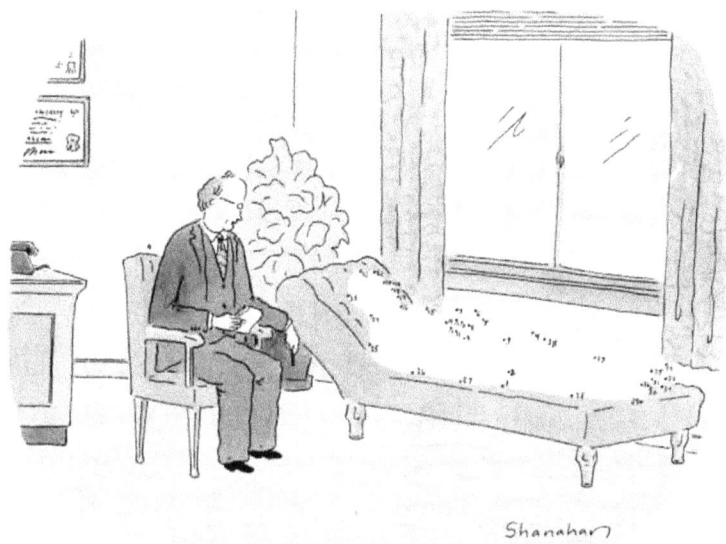

Figure 1: "You've got to want to connect the dots, Mr. Michaelson."

CHAPTER ONE

A New Vision for Our Collective Work

Trauma stewardship is for social workers, ecologists, teachers, firefighters, medical personnel, police officers, environmentalists, home health aides, military personnel, domestic violence workers, biologists, the staffs at animal shelters, international relief workers, social-change activists, those caring for an elderly parent or a young child—in short, anyone who interacts with the suffering, pain, and crisis of others or our planet. It is an approach that applies equally whether the trauma we encounter is glaring or subtle, sudden or prolonged, isolated or recurring, widely recognized or barely perceived. Our stewardship involves but is not limited to our intention in choosing the work we do, our philosophy of what it means to help others, the tone our caregiving takes, and our daily decisions about how we live our life.

Trauma stewardship is not simply an idea. It can be defined as a daily practice through which individuals, organizations, and societies tend to the hardship, pain, or trauma experienced by humans, other living beings, or our planet itself. Those who support trauma stewardship believe that both joy and pain are realities of life, and that suffering can be transformed into meaningful growth and healing when a quality of presence is cultivated and maintained even in the face of great suffering.

Trauma stewardship calls us to engage oppression and trauma—whether through our careers or in our personal lives—by caring for, tending to, and responsibly guiding other beings who are struggling. At the same time, we do not internalize others' struggles or assume them as our own. Trauma stewardship practitioners believe that if we are to alleviate the suffering of others and the planet in the long term, we must respond to even the most urgent human and environmental conditions in a sustainable and intentional way. By developing the deep sense of awareness needed to care for ourselves while caring for others and the world around us, we can greatly enhance our potential to work for change, ethically and with integrity, for generations to come.

The rewards of such a practice are obvious, and it is also a profound challenge. Effective trauma stewardship may require that we question some of our most deeply held beliefs about our lives and work. Many of us might believe, secretly or not so secretly, that our commitment to our work may be measured by our willingness to martyr ourselves. It can be a terrific effort to adopt behaviors or ways of thinking that defy such internal convictions, even when you know the changes are self-respecting, healthy, and entirely necessary.

Because the practice of trauma stewardship demands such a high level of consciousness from us, I feel it's important to lay some groundwork for the process of self-transformation and to explain my intention when I call for a new approach to our collective work.

The most important technique in trauma stewardship is learning to stay fully present in our experience, no matter how difficult. The early American essayist and poet Ralph Waldo Emerson once said, "In skating over thin ice, our safety is in our speed." Our goal is the opposite: When we arrive at a frightening place, we want to slow down enough to be curious about what is happening within ourselves. We want to be "present" with ourselves, an activity that in this book we can consider synonymous with being "mindful." According to Jon Kabat-Zinn, a scientist, author, and educator who has written extensively about the uses of meditation in medicine, mindfulness can be defined as "paying attention in a particular way; on purpose, in the present moment, and non-judgmentally." Daniel Siegel, a doctor, researcher, and educator, describes mindfulness as "being aware of your awareness and paying attention to your intention."

As you begin to observe yourself, be fascinated, intrigued, and in no way critical. Avoid thinking in terms of right or wrong, good or bad, pathological or healthy. As we move away from habitual binary thinking, we can assume an internal posture similar to what a coach might suggest to a runner training for a marathon: chest open, shoulders lowered, jaw relaxed. When we do this, we're more able to go the distance in our self-exploration.

We might phrase our inquiry as follows: If I am exposed to suffering in a single moment or over the arc of time, is there the possibility that I will be affected by such exposure? Like that. No conclusions, no judgment, no defensiveness—just curiosity. We ask, "How am I different now than I was?" Our awakening to some changes may edify us and bring us closer to our values. At moments, our noticing may leave us feeling estranged, angry, or confused. With our tool of curiosity, we can observe the changes in ourselves, our relationships, and our work. The Soto Zen priest Suzuki Roshi said, "All of you are perfect, and you could use a little improvement." (Figure 1.1)

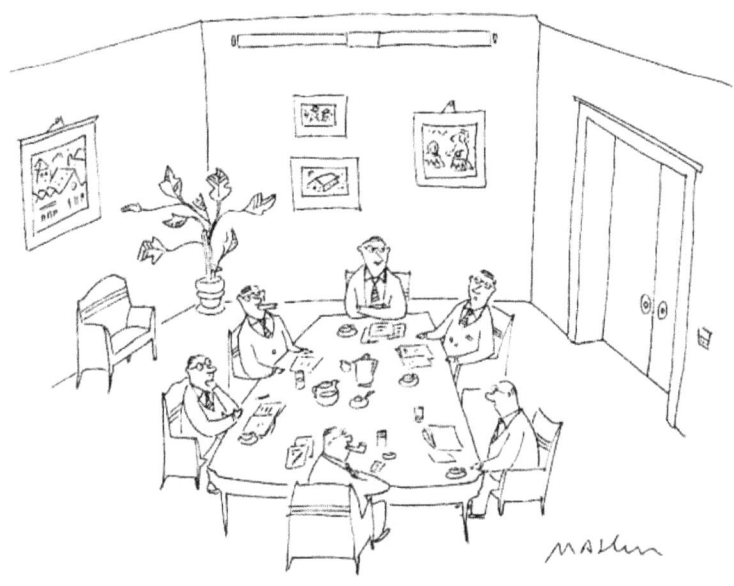

Figure 1.1: "And now at this point in the meeting I'd like to shift the blame away from me and onto someone else."

Maintaining compassion for ourselves and others is of paramount importance as we explore our trauma exposure response. This is the term we use for the wide range of strategies we may have evolved, whether consciously or unconsciously, to contend with the trauma we have witnessed or shared in our lives or our work. We will look closely at these responses in part 2. The more we try to protect ourselves through not being fully present to what is unfolding in our lives, the more we feel the effects of trauma exposure. As you take this in, waste no time in being self-deprecating or in indicting others; be as openhearted and open-minded as you can. When we lose compassion, our capacities to think and feel begin to constrict. If we are going to work optimally on this journey, we will need thinking and feeling in abundance. And the more you can laugh through these chapters, the better.

I encourage you to remember that nothing has to change in the world for us to transform our own life experience. This may be difficult to accept—we may be committed to repairing society on multiple levels, and we may think about our work in relation to large questions of justice, equality, and liberation. We may feel that if we focus on ourselves, we are abandoning our mission. The truth is that we have no authority over many things in our lives, but we do control how we interact with our situation from moment to moment. If we allow our happiness and sense of success to hinge on things outside of ourselves, we will wait for our well-being indefinitely. For example:

"When my boss leaves, I'll feel better." "When we get more funding, things will be smoother." "If I can wrap up my research project, I'll be happier."

Many traditions teach us that regardless of anything external, we can create and re-create how we feel, view the world, and experience our surroundings simply by shifting our perspective. We can ask, "Where am I putting my focus?" If we put aside our fears and simply observe what is in front of us, there is something in every moment to honor. As the Holocaust victim and diarist Anne Frank said, "How wonderful it is that nobody need wait a single moment before starting to improve the world."

Remembering that we have the freedom to choose our path is a central tenet of this book. We are drawing a map that will help us navigate our way to trauma stewardship; the more we understand about where we are, the better our choices about where we go. The first step is to slow down and take stock of where you are now. As you do so, keep in mind that you can decide your course of action with respect to the work you are doing, and resolve to interact with what is in front of you in an honorable way. Intentions like these can go a long way toward sustaining a life of meaning and purpose.

We probably can all identify with the experience of having our friends, our family, or our pets trying to communicate with us about how we've changed, and we probably all know that for any variety of reasons, hearing it from others can create a dynamic of defensiveness or alienation. If we rise to the challenge of becoming aware of our transformation, we'll be acting responsibly not only toward ourselves but toward others. If we've laid the groundwork internally to listen to ourselves with empathy, we may be able to hear others' concerns, feedback, and reflections in a more open way as well.

Although trauma stewardship tells us we have choices about where to put our focus, it does not simply involve putting on a happy face. This approach demands that we embrace a paradox: If we are truly to know joy, we cannot afford to shut down our experience of pain.

We know that there have been many attempts to hide the evidence of suffering in the world. During the Rwandan genocide, Tutsis tried desperately to catch the attention of the international community—but the story was often passed over in favor of less complicated fare. In the aftermath of the killing, many around the globe expressed dismay that people could perpetrate and suffer so much violence without their stories penetrating the consciousness of the world community. It was the question "How could such suffering go unnoticed?" that eventually made the headlines, not the suffering itself.

Many of us who do frontline work to ease trauma and bring about social and environmental change understand that bearing witness, amplifying the story, and taking right action are our most important tasks. But how do we witness, and what is right action? In living out these questions, we often confront choices that leave us feeling anguished and overwhelmed. Which reality should we focus on? Should we focus on the trauma itself? Should we focus on the heroism of women, men, and children who continue to struggle? Should we focus on the economic, environmental, and political practices, past and present, that have created conditions in which violence and destruction thrive? Or should we focus on the amazing capacity of humans to survive, help, love, repent? If we choose wrong—or, worse yet, if our attention strays—how much more suffering will go unnoticed?

The answers to such questions are not easy to find. Even as we struggle to arrive at a usable answer, thornier philosophical questions arise. They are the stuff that has fueled the work of theologians, artists, politicians, healers, poets, and activists for millennia. There are nearly as many theories as there are thinkers about the helper's relationship to those who need help and to the world that created their need.

Of course, too often, suffering does go unnoticed and unattended. Still, people who are working to help those who suffer, or who are working to repair the world to prevent suffering, must somehow reconcile their own joy—the authentic wonder and delight in life—with the irrefutable fact of suffering in the world.

People may come to believe that feeling happy or lighthearted is a betrayal of all of the countless humans, creatures, and environments that are under siege on this planet. They may act as if the only way they can express solidarity with suffering of any kind is by suffering themselves. Even for many well-intentioned, noble, responsible people, the scope of disease, hardship, and pain from the individual to the global level can be overwhelming. People who experience a sense of helplessness may come to believe there is nothing to be done but keep their heads down and hope for the best.

Somewhere between internalizing an ethic of martyrdom and ignoring ongoing crises lies the balance that we must find in order to sustain our work. The more we can attend to this balance, the greater our odds of achieving a sustainable practice of trauma stewardship.

My work for trauma stewardship starts with each of us as individuals. This emphasis comes from my personal belief, rooted in life experience and years of study and professional practice, that our capacity to help others and the environment is greatest when we are willing, able, and even determined to be helped ourselves. As Gandhi, the political and spiritual leader of India and its independence movement, said, "Be the change you want to see in the world."

When I say that each of us should take responsibility for becoming trauma stewards, however, I do not mean that any of us is in this alone. This book does not propose a "pull yourself up by your own bootstraps" approach to coping with the effects of exposure to trauma. Our ability to function as effective trauma stewards is directly influenced by the organizations we work for, as well as by the systems and attitudes that prevail in society at large. Every larger system has an obligation to the people who make it work, as well as to the people it serves. (Figure 1.2)

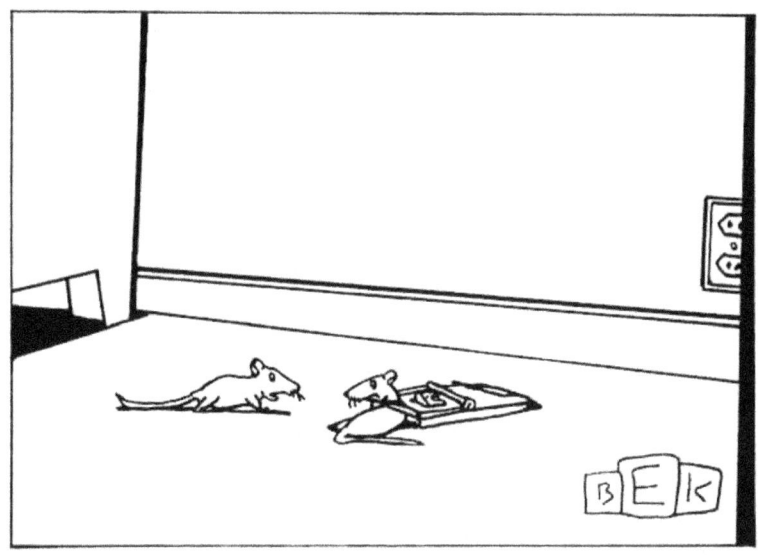

Figure 1.2: "I'm sorry—here I am going on and on and I haven't asked you a thing about being caught in a trap."

At the same time, each of us must recognize that we have a role to play in shaping the organizations and social systems we participate in. Trauma always creates a ripple effect, the same as when someone throws a stone into a still pond. The initial impact creates repercussions that expand almost infinitely, reaching and having an effect on many people who didn't experience the blows firsthand. The shockwaves soon move beyond individual caregivers to influence the organizations and systems in which we work and, ultimately, the society as a whole. The harms of trauma exposure response radiate in this way, but so do the benefits of trauma stewardship.

Like individuals, organizations and institutions may unwittingly respond to trauma exposure in ways that prevent them from fully realizing their mission to help. Lacking the resources and means to realize their goals, they can actually increase their clients' distress and create hardship for workers.

The same is true on the societal level. Larger systems may also contribute to suffering even as they attempt to alleviate it. In the United States, we see this dynamic in examples as diverse as the health care industry and the justice system. The health care industry is intended to limit suffering but instead often winds up magnifying trauma exposure for patients, their workers, and the organizations that interact with them. Similarly, cooperating with law enforcement or testifying in court may inadvertently increase the anguish of crime victims. Reflecting on the lessons of my own extensive experience in organizations, I have come to realize that sometimes I was a part of the problem even as I aspired to be part of the solution.

This can be difficult to acknowledge; as workers, we may have a lot invested in these systems. But as we explore trauma stewardship, we must be willing to recognize that there are major flaws in our organizations, institutions, and societal systems—and that these shortcomings affect us and the way we do our jobs. We will talk more about the three levels of trauma stewardship in the next chapter. Although a complete exploration of the organizational and societal ramifications of our work is beyond the scope of this book, all of our discussions of personal change are intended to take place in the context of this larger framework.

If we are to contribute to the changes so desperately needed in our agencies, communities, and societies, we must first and foremost develop the capacity to be present with all that arises, stay centered throughout, and be skilled at maintaining an integrated self. For many, this requires a daily practice of "handling your business," as the singer and social activist Stevie Wonder says. Our goal is to reach the places where we can conduct our own lives with ethics and integrity—day after day, and in situation after situation. The more that we can accomplish this, the clearer our path at every level of trauma stewardship will be.

CHAPTER TWO

The Three Levels of Trauma Stewardship

> The rule of no realm is mine, neither Gondor nor any other, great or small. But all worthy things that are in peril as the world now stands, those are my care. And for my part, I shall not wholly fail in my task, though Gondor should perish, if anything that passes through this night can still grow fairer or bear fruit and flower again in days to come. For I too am a steward. Did you not know?
>
> Gandalf, in J.R.R. Tolkien's *Lord of the Rings: The Return of the King*

In the following pages, we will consider some of the specific ways in which suffering may be perpetuated at the individual, organizational, and societal levels. Reactions to the hardships of humans, animals, and our planet—that is, trauma exposure response—may manifest very differently at each of these three levels, but the risk of behaviors that inadvertently magnify the pain and suffering of direct trauma is always present. The more deeply we realize this, the more we understand the potential—and the necessity—for a trauma stewardship approach. I encourage you to keep all three levels in mind as you read this book. If we can transform ourselves, we have the potential to change the world.

Personal Dynamics

One of the most profound influences on trauma stewardship is who we are as individuals. What is our own history of hardship, pain, suffering, and trauma? What resources were available to help us? What led us to the work we do? The more personal our connection to our work, the greater the gifts we bring to it—perhaps. At the same time, the more we identify with the type of trauma we're exposed to, the greater its impact on us may be. (Figure 2.1)

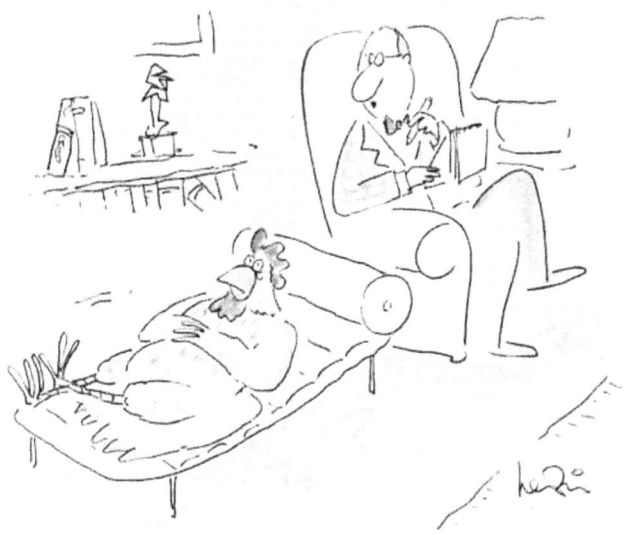

Figure 2.1: "Why do you think you cross the road?"

Prison work will have a different impact on someone who has never been incarcerated or had a friend or relative in prison than on someone who lives in a community where 40 percent of the men are currently incarcerated. If you have no personal history linking you to your work, you may be able to care deeply about it while still maintaining some useful distance from it. This distance may limit your insights about your work, but you may retain greater reserves of psychic strength if you are not also reexperiencing the pain of familiar wounds.

On the other hand, if you are working with a population with whom you have a history, you may feel a rawness as you approach your work. This rawness may allow you to connect with the work in an intimate, knowing way. Although we can never presume to fully understand what it's like to walk in another's shoes, you may indeed have a very good sense of what that walk feels like, looks like, sounds like, and tastes like. While this awareness may help guide you, it also can dramatically heighten your own vulnerabilities as someone who can truly feel the other's pain.

For many workers, it is difficult to perceive a clear line between the personal and the professional. Obviously, this is not the case for everyone whose work and personal history overlap, but there is often a correlation. To be an effective trauma steward, it is important to know where our own self ends and another's self begins. This can be a hard distinction to maintain even when we are working with other adults, who, whatever their difficulties, are clearly separate people with agency in their own lives. Ironically, it may be even more challenging when we are working with populations that seem particularly defenseless—young children, for example, or abused animals or endangered species. When we speak up for people or creatures or environments that are unable to speak for themselves, we may gradually lose the ability to distinguish their voices from our own. If we don't pay careful attention, our feelings of identification and responsibility may increase to the point that we experience their anguish in a debilitating way. In the long run, this can diminish our ability to be effective advocates. We can sustain our work with trauma only if we combine our capacity for empathy with a dedication to personal insight and mindfulness. This is difficult terrain to navigate.

Organizational Tendencies

I honestly think every person I work with in my division is on antidepressants at this point ... everyone here.
Child protective services caseworker

Organizations play a multifaceted role in trauma stewardship. The people who make up any organization help to shape its culture, so in some ways each organization is a reflection of the collective capacity for trauma stewardship of all the individuals involved. At the same time, organizations themselves have the potential to either mitigate or exacerbate the effects of trauma exposure for all of their workers. The way those workers manage trauma will in turn have an impact on the experiences of already traumatized clients. Golie Jansen, an associate professor at Eastern Washington University, recently concluded a study in which she found that "when people perceive their organizations to be supportive, they experience lower levels of vicarious trauma."

Because of multiple and conflicting objectives, insufficient resources, and other difficulties, organizations often ask employees and/or volunteers to perform demanding jobs without adequate support. As a result, people are unable to do their jobs as well as they would like. For example, many teachers in the United States find themselves unable to attend to their students' emotional needs—an essential element of creating a good learning environment—and at the same time prepare them for the rigorous state exams required by the No Child Left Behind legislation. Doctors are unable to attend to the psychosocial needs of their patients because they work for medical organizations that limit the time for each patient visit. (Figure 2.2)

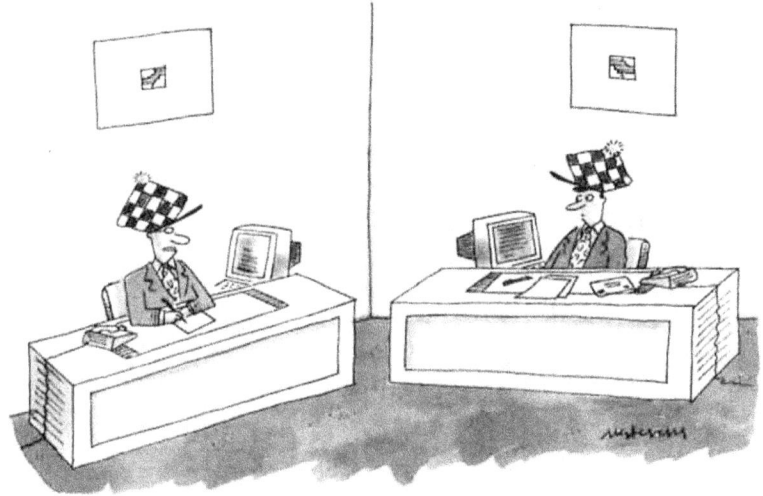

Figure 2.2: "I don't know bow it started, either. All I know is that it's part of our corporate culture."

This leads to a phenomenon that Michael Lipsky, a political scientist and the author of *Street-Level Bureaucracy,* calls *service rationing.* Service rationing refers to the process that workers go through to bridge the everyday divide between the ideal of how they *would* work if they were free to function to the best of their ability and the reality of how they *can* work, given the numerous obstacles in their way. An effect of service rationing is the continual defining and redefining of one's job. If it's not quite the work you had originally hoped to do, you mentally redefine it in some way that allows you to reconcile the growing contradiction.

How much these cognitive shifts are necessary varies from organization to organization, policy to policy, and supervisor to supervisor. Still, many workers walk a common path, trying to find a satisfactory compromise between what they can do and what they are asked to do. Service rationing surfaces when a legal aid attorney is more sympathetic to a compliant client who seems willing to take direction than to one who is belligerent, for example, or when a homeless shelter worker prioritizes the resident talking loudly about suicidal fantasies over the resident who is morose but just as severely depressed.

Initially, many workers may find that these choices go deeply against the grain. They truly want to attend to everyone equally. But over time, rationalizing such behavior may be the only way to contain remorse and preserve a sense of satisfaction in your work. A social worker in the Office of Indian Child Welfare who is in the 28th year of her career told me, "I had three supervisors in one year and a coworker who committed suicide. I was so overloaded that I had to figure out, given my caseload, what the bare minimum was that I could do while continuing to serve my clients well and trying to not get in trouble myself."

Service rationing is paradoxical. It may diminish people's spirits and possibly the quality of their work, but at the same time it is often an essential coping mechanism. Without it, many people simply couldn't stay in their jobs at all. As we can see from Lipsky's research, there is a desperate need for environments that help people to do good work and achieve personal satisfaction even when compromises are inevitable. Without effective policy in place, both direct service delivery and efforts at larger social change are undermined. Ethical work cannot be sustained in an eroding environment that fails to support its workers.

Lipsky also coined the phrase *street-level bureaucrat.* This is a neutral term that describes many police officers, lower court judges, social workers, and countless other public service workers. It refers not to their personalities but to the characteristics of their work. Street-level bureaucrats are workers who interact with people in ways that significantly affect the clients' lives, who have broad decision-making power with respect to these interactions, and who lack sufficient resources to do their job the best they can. Furthermore, they are in positions where it is hard to hold them accountable because of the wide discretion they have in their jobs.

Some street-level bureaucrats do their jobs ethically and well, hold their heads high, and find satisfaction in their efforts. Others may become defeated by their work, make poor choices, and shirk their responsibilities. Street-level bureaucrats are prime candidates to adopt service rationing as a coping mechanism. Facing overwhelming challenges, they salvage job satisfaction by shooting for lowered goals that they have some hope of meeting. A high school math teacher with too many students may seek professional gratification by focusing on the most advanced pupils, who are more likely to be boys; as a result, the girls, who often begin to lag in math and science after receiving less encouragement in their middle school years, may not get the attention they need to catch up. In the long run, such coping mechanisms add up to policies detrimental to society.

Good policy, both political and personal, takes into account the reality of the need for service rationing. Effective policymakers look without flinching at the possibility that scarcity of resources will require workers to take shortcuts. We should strive for policy that eliminates the need for shortcuts—and, if they are unavoidable, tries to preserve results that are as close as possible to what we want as a society.

Our responses to trauma exposure can foster a defended, exclusive, and hopeless culture in the organizations we work for. Think about how your workplace feels. What's the energy level? What's the vibe? These qualities have nothing to do with the intensity of the work. Instead, they have to do with the degree to which the organization's structures, policies, and attitudes support or impede the workers' efforts to fulfill the mission.

In the early days of HIV/AIDS in Seattle, there was an organization (still around as of this writing) called People of Color Against AIDS Network. This was one of the most exquisite places I had ever encountered, and every time I left the building, I couldn't wait to go back. The work was intense, difficult, and often very sad, but the feeling we had working together was amazing. There were people who were radiant, who sang while they worked, who took time to catch up daily on each other's families, who lovingly greeted everyone with whom they came in contact, who remained inspired in spite of the despair around them.

And then there were other organizations whose buildings I left desperate to take a shower and rid myself of the feeling I had experienced just being there. It wasn't about the condition of the carpet or how many multicultural posters were on the walls. It was whether light and hope and feelings of possibility were emanating from the institution or whether the organizational culture felt negative, exclusive, and hopeless. There are many factors affecting organizational culture. The negative ones range from irrational norms to ineffective leadership to nonsensical personnel policies.

A longtime leader in the domestic violence movement, Beth Richie, recounts a story illustrating how organizational culture can become confused over time. During a visit to a confidential domestic violence shelter for women and children, she happened to overhear one of the advocates preventing a child from taking a banana off the kitchen counter. The advocate said, "Oh no, I'm sorry, the bananas are not for the children." It was an eerie moment, Richie said. An organization's culture can become so steeped in notions of scarcity that it enforces policies radically incongruent with the original mission.

We frequently see trauma exposure response manifest in our work in two other ways: lack of accountability and unethical behavior. A *New York Times Magazine* article in 2000 told the story of Kerry Sanders, a man with a history of mental illness who was arrested for sleeping on a park bench, mistaken in court for a fugitive with the same last name, and sent to prison, where he served two years for a crime he had never committed. The article traced the progression of this horrendous story from the police to the mental health workers to the prison guards to the probation workers to the attorneys and so on. Ultimately, over 20 professionals were deposed to try to make some sense of how this had occurred and why Sanders had spent years in prison unjustly.

No decent answers were found. From prosecutor to prison guard to recreational therapist to psychiatrist to nurse, everyone claimed they were blameless. They replied to Sanders' pleas for help with a range of responses from "I let him know there was nothing I could do" to "I am not a legal aid society" to "It's not my job—I don't do that." The article described how "a prison psychiatrist who treated Mr. Sanders said that given his mental problems and homelessness, he was better off in prison. 'He should say, "Thank you, for two years you guys treated me very nicely."'"

The article concluded, "The issues of responsibility and culpability, of quality of care and of monumental and systematic failings, continue to surround the lawsuit. Yet in 2,000 pages of depositions, there have been few displays of compassion and fewer of outrage. At Green Haven [the prison where Sanders was held], no one on the staff was even told what happened, and no one asked. One day, Kerry Sanders just disappeared."

In almost every paragraph of the article is an example of how a trauma exposure response, on both the individual and organizational levels, was a contributing factor in the lack of accountability and the unethical behavior that led to the incarceration of an innocent man. This is partially a testament to the power of denial and rationalization as they relate to unethical behavior; I imagine the people involved in this story truly believed on some level that they were not to blame. A follow-up article the next year quoted a New York correctional services spokesman, James B. Flateau, as saying, "The commissioner's feeling was that as unfortunate as the outcome was, there was no venality on the part of any employees. It was just an incredible confluence of events that we had never before seen happen." Robert Gangi, executive director of the Correctional Association of New York, a prison monitoring group, said, "It's definitely a worst-case kind of scenario, and at the same time it reflects the lack of attention and lack of resources that the state devotes to prison mental health services."

Often, people begin recognizing the effect of trauma exposure when they realize they are behaving in ways they never would have when they first started working in their field. Perhaps when workers start out, they have the energy required to navigate the gray areas of their work, to question their assumptions, to stay open-minded about what is possible, and to truly believe that it matters if they do right in the work and in the world. Over time, the complexity of the issues may surface, the scarcity of resources may feel overwhelming, and one may feel more and more isolated. At that point, a sense of entitlement creeps in: We may feel so desperate for satisfaction that we will try to meet the clients' needs by any means necessary—and so what if it compromises the integrity of the work? After all, who is going to notice? Who is going to care?

The vast majority of people I've worked with are not stealing office supplies or embezzling money. Instead, just as in the examples above, they may be unknowingly abusing their power in their client interactions, or developing policies that are not mindful and consistent with the values of the organization, or competing with other organizations instead of collaborating. In my experience, when this type of behavior takes root, born out of some of the reasons we discussed above, it can become a tremendous source of guilt. Later on, when we survey the specific aspects of a trauma exposure response and how they surface in our lives, we'll see that guilt, fatigue, a sense of entitlement, and other deeply ingrained habits are all facets of the same cumulative effect.

Societal Forces

To fully comprehend trauma stewardship, we must pull our perspective back even more. We want to understand how society at large interfaces with our trauma exposure response. If we are ever to realize our hopes of creating and re-creating a society in which we are all free from suffering, we must take a macro view.

Without a sense of the big picture, it is impossible to have any meaningful conversation about what we want to do collectively to improve the circumstances of our lives and work.

We can use the analogy of cleaning up a river. Retrieving and recycling the plastic bottles or other debris we find floating toward us is a needed step in a cleanup. But to be stewards, more is required. We can't just pick up trash and dig out polluted sediments at the stretch of river directly in front of us. We need to identify and address all the sources of that pollution. We start with the local community, asking people to stop littering or dumping household chemicals down the drain. Beyond that, we need to go upstream. We need to look for factories piping chemicals to the river, septic systems leaking contaminants to its banks, and polluted rainwater as it runs off a hundred roadways to contaminate a dozen tributaries. We need to look to the sky, where the toxic emissions produced by distant coal plants fall from the air as acid rain. To do the cleanup right and to make sure that it lasts, we need to foster a stronger sense of conservation in the citizens and businesses of an entire region. Trauma stewardship works much the same way. Numerous forces contribute to the flow of trauma, and to accomplish lasting repair, we need shifts in attitudes and practices by ourselves, our organizations, and our infrastructures, thus protecting the watershed for years to come.

Rooting our concept of trauma stewardship in a larger framework of systematic oppression and liberation theory is extremely important. Oppression plays a leading role in creating and maintaining systems that perpetuate suffering and trauma for all sentient beings, as well as the planet we share. The more we can understand this relationship, the better our insights into the ways that trauma affects us individually and collectively around the globe.

Oppression can be defined as the negative outcome experienced by people who are targeted by the cruel exercise of power; the term is generally used to describe how a certain group is being kept down by unjust use of authority, force, or societal norms. When a society institutionalizes oppression formally or informally, the result is called *systematic oppression.* Around the globe, liberation movements promote the undoing of negative outcomes and the elimination of the causes of individual and systematic oppression.

In recent decades, many liberationist thinkers have made their voices heard in indigenous and diaspora freedom movements, as well as in environmental justice movements worldwide. Examples include Father Gustavo Gutiérrez, a Peruvian Catholic priest and liberation theologist; the late Paulo Freire, a Brazilian educator; Rigoberta Menchú Tum, a Guatemalan advocate of indigenous land rights and winner of the Nobel Peace Prize; Reverend Allan Aubrey Boesak, a South African anti-apartheid activist and theologian; and Vandana Shiva, an Indian biophysicist and environmental ethicist. There are many others.

One example of systematic oppression is *structural violence.* This concept was introduced in the 1970s by Johan Galtung, a pioneering Norwegian researcher in peace and conflict, and founder of the International Peace Research Institute. He describes structural violence as "a form of violence which corresponds with the systematic ways in which a given social structure or social institution kills people slowly by preventing them from meeting their basic needs. Institutionalized elitism, ethnocentricism, classism, racism, sexism, adultism, nationalism, heterosexism and ageism are just some examples of structural violence. Life spans are reduced when people are socially dominated, politically oppressed, or economically exploited. Structural violence and direct violence are highly interdependent. Structural violence inevitably produces conflict and often direct violence including family violence, racial violence, hate crimes, terrorism, genocide, and war." Paul Farmer, an American medical anthropologist and founder of the international health and social justice organization Partners In Health, elaborates: "Structural violence is visited upon all those whose social status denies them access to the fruits of scientific and social progress." (Figure 2.3)

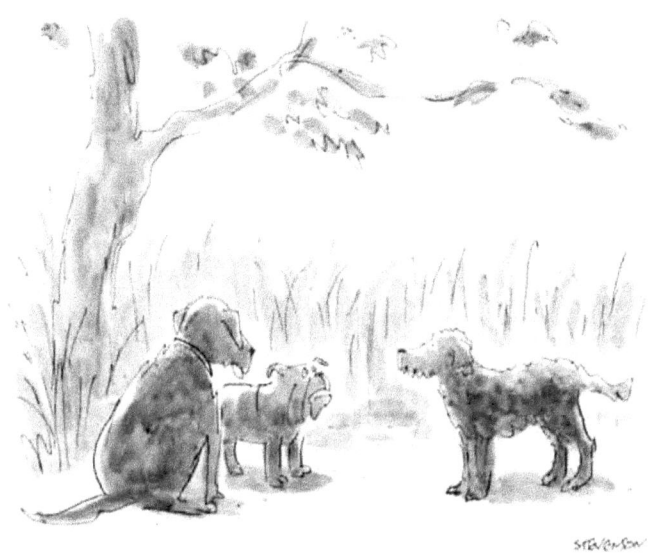

Figure 2.3: "Speaking personally, I haven't had my day, and Pve never met any doe who has."

If we lived in a society where equity, respect, access, and justice were realized, and unearned privilege and inequality and oppression were transformed, the impact of trauma exposure in our lives would look dramatically different. Suffering would still occur. People would sustain injuries and contract illnesses and even hurt each other. The difference is that we would only have to confront that suffering at face value: an injury, an illness, a hurtful act. We would not have to wonder if disparities between rich and poor, white people and people of color, heterosexual people and gay/lesbian/bi/transgendered people, and so on contributed to the suffering. We would not have to wonder if we personally benefit from the disparity that underlies the suffering. We would not have to wonder if we are vulnerable to the same disparity. We would not have to decide whether we should act to change the disparity, or if we should blame the person suffering for the disparity, or if we should ignore the disparity altogether.

In this ideal society, people would respond to our work differently as well. If, when you told others what you did, they stopped, looked you in the eye, thanked you, and offered to make a donation, the impact of your work would look very different than it does now. If we feel that it's consistently a conversation stopper, or if we believe we have to lie about what we do because so many people don't understand it, or if we perceive that others constantly judge us when they express disgust about our work or make objectifying comments like, "You're such an a-n-g-e-l! I could never do that job!" the toll of our work is that much higher.

We can see an example of that toll when we look at those who attend to our elders. "Caregiver stress is directly related to the way our society views the elderly and the people who care for them," elder-care expert Vitaliano says in the LeRoy article on CNN.com cited in the introduction. The text continues: "Today, caregiving is viewed largely as a burden in this country. If it were viewed as more of a societal expectation and people were willing to offer more support, fewer caregivers would suffer in isolation, [Vitaliano] says. In turn, fewer elder and disabled people would experience abuse or neglect at the hands of caregiving individuals or institutions."

The researchers and trauma experts Bessel A. van der Kolk and Alexander C. McFarlane write, "Reason and objectivity are not the primary determinants of society's reactions to traumatized people. Rather ... society's reactions seem to be primarily conservative impulses in the service of maintaining the beliefs that the world is fundamentally just, that people can be in charge of their lives, and that bad things only happen to people who deserve them."

I have frequently seen such irrational and defensive "conservative impulses" applied to organizational systems over the years, but perhaps never more than when I have collaborated with child protective services (CPS) workers and firefighters. Both groups have grueling, scary, demanding jobs, and yet the way people react to them is strikingly different. CPS workers carry a heavy burden of feeling that they are hated—by everyone. Firefighters, on the other hand, tend to have the benefit of an age-old image of them as saviors and heroes. This contrast speaks to every level we've touched on: the personal, the organizational, and the societal.

There are several underpinnings to this discussion of systematic oppression. Oppression thrives on misunderstanding, alienation, and us/them binaries. Many people have judgments about those who are hurt, raped, sick, addicted, and so on, and as a result, people are often uncomfortable when we tell them what we do. The way people act toward us in response to our work makes the impact of trauma exposure more profound because it increases our sense of isolation, and isolation is one of the staples that keeps systematic oppression firmly in place. Of course, we participate in sustaining this dynamic of isolation ourselves—for example, when we avoid speaking about our work because we fear it will initiate a debate we don't have the energy to engage in, when we lie about what we do because we believe that others will not understand, when we react defensively because we expect other people's comments to be judgmental or dismissive, or even when we, in a particular field, keep to ourselves because we anticipate that our work—with families in the suburbs, with abandoned animals, or with endangered ecosystems—will be derided as diverting resources from more urgent human service needs.

We are hardly alone in avoiding potentially troubling interactions. In the book *Traumatic Stress,* van der Kolk and McFarlane write that "individuals, and even entire cultures, build up elaborate defenses in order to keep these stark realities out of conscious awareness." In writing these chapters, I have tried to begin a weakening of these defenses. This overview aims to alert you to the far-reaching consequences of trauma exposure response and to its effects on trauma stewardship. I am drawing the atlas for a terrain that you already inhabit, although you may not know exactly where. In a sense, I have sketched out the borders of a large country—and in part 2, I will provide you with the information you may need to determine exactly what state you are in.

PROFILE CINDY PARRY

THE OZARKS, RURAL MISSOURI
CURRENTLY: Clinical resource manager for Air Evac Lifeteam, an emergency helicopter service for rural America, with 68 bases.
FORMERLY: Paramedic, nurse (emergency room, post-anesthesia

care, and flight), childbirth educator, community activist.

I was fine. I mean, I was tired of taking care of sick people. It was always best for me when they were intubated and paralyzed and couldn't talk at all ... so ... Well, so I guess it was time for me to get out.

Here's the deal. When I first got into the paramedic field, I was one of a very few women in the profession, and I think that made a difference in the attitude that was out there. The attitude was, if you can't take the heat, get out of the kitchen. The critical incident stress debriefing, or recognizing a normal response to an abnormal event, was just starting to come around; there was not much consciousness about a trauma exposure response. You just toughed it out, and if you weren't able to deal with it, then you needed to get another job. You just quit.

I can clearly remember the day and the specific call when I had had enough. I was like, "That's enough, I'm done." I realized then how it had impacted me. You see so much, and there are certain things that get revisited that still come up, certain situations and calls, and I remember this one so clearly. We'd gone to a motorcycle accident, and as you approached the scene, it was clear he was dead and he was in several pieces, his body. I had this long-standing irritation with my paramedic partner about his leaving his belongings all over the place when we worked. I was always having to clean up after him. So at this accident, for some reason I thought it'd be funny to take his camera from the ambulance and take photos of this motorcycle accident so that when he developed his film, he'd come across these photos. I was clicking these pictures, and I thought it was a great joke. And a couple of days later I thought, "You know what, maybe I need to do something else."

It wasn't that I could not do my job, because I did it extremely well, partly because I could get totally disconnected from what I had to do.

And I saw those people who'd been doing it a while, and I thought, "I don't want to be like those people; those people are assholes." This motorcycle accident was the turning point for me. It wasn't necessarily the bloodiest or the worst accident I'd worked on, but the fact that I could start taking pictures with my partner's camera and the fact that that would be a big joke to me—it was like, how the hell could you do that? I mean, that is just sick.

After quitting being a paramedic, I moved to southern Missouri, which is a place where it's really hard to make a living unless you have a portable skill. I intended to train as a midwife, but instead I got back into this emergency medicine thing. That is what I knew how to do, so I finished up my bachelor's degree and took care of my dying mom while going through nursing school. I thought I'd do anything but the ER, but then there's something about the ER that I just love. There's something very compelling about it. I like the variety of what you see. It's real. It's amazing to save a life. I mean, my God, it's just totally amazing. When you feel like you've had an impact in a big way, that a person wouldn't be alive, and not only just alive but recovered, and you've had a big part in that, that's pretty compelling.

One of the ways I've been impacted by my work is I just view everything as a head injury waiting to happen. I'm a lot less callous about things. I'm much more aware of how fragile everything is. [At Air Evac Lifeteam, where she works now] part of what I do is read through flight records, and with some of the more dramatic calls I think, "This is the day the person's life changed forever, this family's life changed forever." I am much more aware of the impact that has on people. It's so easy to slip back into the "You're just dealing with the broken arm," the compartmentalizing. It's a struggle to keep a consciousness that you're dealing with human beings and not just dealing with body parts, and it's a struggle to be present on all the levels you need to be for people and their families.... Ohhh, I hate the families. It's so easy to check out and just fix the thing that's broken. I'm aware that I need to have my whole self present, but it's so hard to do.

Most of the people who survive and go on and who are people I want to be like are people who keep their whole selves there while doing this work. I guess that's about compassion in some way.

What's hard about the families is that feeling of "Don't bother me anymore" that I have. In the ER and the ICU and the critical care and I'm sure any nursing thing, there are constant demands on you. You've got to do your job, which more and more is paperwork and reports. So with the families, they're just a pain in the ass ... they keep you from getting these things done. We used to joke to remind ourselves that the patient's the point and not the problem. We'd joke that it'd be a really great job if it wasn't for all these pesky patients.

The other thing is control, control, control. I want control and the patients want control and the families want information and want to be in control, too. There's been this whole evolution of nursing being more overloaded and things being crappier. I think part is the overload from administrators, part is from the health care system, part is from the direct patient care.

It sounds trite, but I'm more appreciative of things now than I ever was before. It's always amazing to me what the human body can sustain. Like, I love skin. Skin is an amazing thing. How can you be so broken and you don't even have a cut on you? It's always just so puzzling, and there's the great mystery: What the hell will kill you is the little thing, and what won't kill you is the hugest thing. Someone is walking, trips, and they're dead. Then a car goes off a cliff and that person survives. The randomness of life is mysterious, and as much control as you want to have over things, you just don't have any control over shit, and in a way that's not frightening. I used to think that was scary, but in a way it's not. You can be as careful as you can be and then a bale of hay can fall on you and kill you. And so you realize you don't have any control. You really don't. You can lose it in a flash. I have such impatience with whining. With friends and with myself. I think, for God's sake, you don't even know how lucky you are.

What helps me keep on keeping on is that I don't do direct patient care anymore. Also therapy, man. I don't think I'm particularly sane. I don't think I've always been able to be so balanced. I put my hands in dirt. And I have the most amazing drive into work. Forty-five minutes of some of the most spectacular and beautiful scenery. When you see the mist come up from the river and you see the sun come up and you think, "Holy crap, look where I am," and if that's the way you're starting out your day as you go into work, it puts things in perspective. Being able to be outside and connected with things that are so much bigger than I am. I have a great community and a connection with the outdoors. I've got to be out there. Even in my home there's a very thin wall between me and the outside, literally.

I decided to change jobs five months ago [when she left her direct patient care work and took an administrative job with Air Evac]. I was just tired. I thought I'd miss it. I loved the people I worked with in the post-anesthesia care. They say that's where critical care nurses go to die. I loved the women that I worked with. They were so smart and funny and so good at what they did, and I learned so much from them. It was like hanging out with your friends all day. But I just got tired of taking care of people. And I was physically tired. Sometimes I feel drawn to be a flight nurse again on the helicopter, but then it's raining out or really cold, and I get some horrible call. Because we're in such a rural area and because of some crazy thing that happened, those people are out there with their asses literally hanging out of the helicopter and they're having to make these life-and-death decisions. I'm thinking, "Thank God it's not me." What I miss is not patient care. I miss the camaraderie of being with my friends. Sometimes I miss that adrenaline-junkie state of "Damn, didn't we do a good job?" The kick is that you take chaos and you make order out of it, and I miss that. But I don't miss taking care of sick people.

I remember when I first thought about getting into emergency medicine. I was in Colorado at a Girl Scout retreat, and we were in the mountains and there was a lightning strike and the airlift came in to get someone, and I thought, "Cool, I could do that. That could be fun." And so I did. It's been a blast. In looking back about why I got into it, it makes sense. I like to have control, and I like to fix things. And for not a very good or healthy reason I was really able to compartmentalize, to separate.

I would say that my ability to dissociate got stronger. Sometimes that breaks down, though, that ruptures.

I don't know what triggered it, but when I took on this new job at Air Evac Life, things came back to me. I thought, "Wow, look at this again." I remember being at the site of a car accident, and there was a young boy who was maybe 16, and this kid has stuck with me forever. It was some stupid thing, the accident, I don't remember what had happened, but he was dead when we got there. We worked on him anyway, but he was dead. The mother showed up on the scene, and as we were zipping him into a body bag I remember her screams—just that grief, you know that grief—and I looked up to the sky and it was an absolutely gorgeous night. It was a dark, clear sky with beautiful stars, and I remember thinking, "How can these things exist at the same time?"

That was 15 years ago, and I have carried that guy around with me. I knew I did, but to have it come back again was a shock. And I have carried his mother around with me, too. She turned up at the ER later with a picture of her son to show us. I remember thinking, "Man, I do not want to be here right now. I do not want to deal with you." And then years later she comes back to me and becomes fresh again. We were just looking at a slide show of different accidents, and they came back. I remember this 18-month-old and I still see him in his little train pajamas, and his mom was eight months pregnant. I remember her arriving at the hospital, I was feeling so absolutely helpless, and what do you say to them? I couldn't do it. I could not save your child. Sorry.

It's always those damn parents that come back to you. You think they're gone, but I think those things will stay forever. So I wonder, what does this mean? I mean, what happened with that family? If anything happened to one of my kids or my grandson, you'd just have to carry me around in a basket ... it'd be the end of my life. The thing about the rural-area work is everyone's related. I remember a pregnant woman and her mother and some other relative of theirs were brought into the ER at the same time. Even though they did an emergency C-section, the new baby was dead, the mama was dead and the other woman was dead, and then the husband walks in, and you just have to tell him that all your female relatives are dead. How the hell do you do that?

I think I'm letting go of the dissociation. There's some part of you that you have to separate a little in order to do your job. You have to focus on what you're doing, but I think you don't have to separate entirely, and I think I've gotten better at doing this. You know, it's kind of sad, because there is some part of me that thinks we really need our experienced people. We need to be able to keep those experienced nurses that know so much, and we're just burning them out. I have gotten to a point where I am able to bring all these aspects into my job, but I'm too tired to do my job anymore. I am finally able to recognize that we might not be able to stuff things down and go on, and that maybe we could keep people in the field longer and healthier if there were a way to deal with feelings and not be labeled as weak, crazy, or whatever else. It doesn't mean I won't go do it somewhere else, the third world or somewhere in the Ozarks, but not in the hospital, not in the ER. Or maybe you could do it for 4 hours at a time, but you sure as hell can't do it for 12 hours anymore.

It's like you have to have some degree of separation to do some of the typical things that you do, but you just don't have to view everybody as a body part, and I think with either getting older or being in the business as long as I have, I've made it a conscious effort to bring more compassion to what I'm doing. I don't know that it starts out with the big things like the emergency code or the trauma that comes into the ER. It's more the frequent-flyer person that wants to check into the psych ward, and it's just like, "For God's sake," because you know they're going to jam up the ER. You know you aren't going to find a bed, and then you're going to be stuck with this loon all night, and they're going to generate a lot of paperwork which you don't have time to do. I don't know what happened, but I realized that this person did not just say, "You know what, I think it'd be really fun to go to the ER, to be stuck there all night freaking out and to be humiliated and to know that no one wants to deal with me; that is how I want to spend my Friday night."

I am just having a little more awareness. Something clicked for me. I have compassion now for those people. Sometimes you get caught by things, and I got caught by that. By that realization of what it means to be more compassionate.

PART TWO

Mapping Your Response to Trauma Exposure

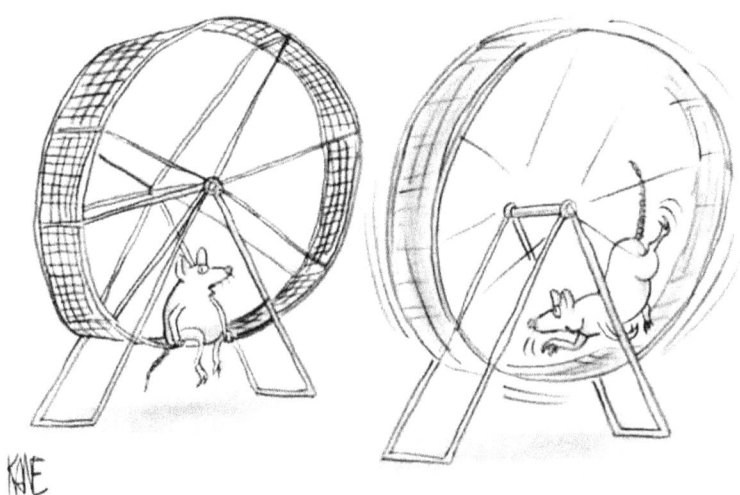

Figure 2: "I had an cpiphany."

CHAPTER THREE

What Is Trauma Exposure Response?

> It was not until last week, after being gone months and after going and picking herbs day after day and making tinctures, that I could think again like myself. It really scared me because I wasn't sure I was going to ever come back.
>
> Mo O'Brien, a street medic who helped create one of the first medical clinics in New Orleans after Hurricane Katrina

If we are to do our work with suffering people and environments in a sustainable way, we must understand how our work affects us. We need to undertake an honest assessment of how our feelings or behaviors have changed in response to whatever trauma we have been exposed to. Generally speaking, a trauma exposure response may be defined as the transformation that takes place within us as a result of exposure to the suffering of other living beings or the planet. This transformation can result from deliberate or inadvertent exposure, formal or informal contact, paid or volunteer work. When we refer to trauma exposure response, we are talking about the ways in which the world looks and feels like a different place to you as a result of your doing your work.

Because trauma exposure hits so close to home for so many people working in helping professions, it can be hard not to feel defensive or overwhelmed when learning about it. Acknowledging the presence of a trauma exposure response means recognizing that things are definitely *not* how we'd like them to be in our lives. In most cases, if we hope to alleviate the situation, change must occur on a fundamental level. For someone already stressed to her or his limit, this can be frightening or feel like an impossible task.

Evaluating our response to trauma exposure is critical, because how we are impacted by our work in the present directly affects our work in the future. Our relationship with our work influences our inner life as well as our experiences with others. It can set in motion a cycle of damage that, if not for our awareness, can overtake our whole lives.

A trauma exposure response has occurred when external trauma becomes internal reality. When this happens as a result of our work, it can catch us off guard. Indeed, the thought that the pain around us can actually change our own psychological and physiological responses, altering our worldview, may never have occurred to us. We often assume that our very status as helpers grants us immunity from the suffering we witness. We are often wrong.

Laurie Leitch, a researcher, educator, and cofounder of the Trauma Resource Institute, which specializes in the impact of trauma on the nervous system, went to work in Thailand after the 2004 tsunami. She was struck by how many workers arrived in a "heroic mode," in which they were exceptionally open to those they had come to help. "As you care for people with your heart wide open, you often don't realize how much of what you are exposed to is being taken in and held in your body. It isn't until later that your body starts to let you know. I thought I was fine over there, until I got home and had nightmares, headaches, and was so irritable. We need to appreciate the impact of humanitarian work not just on the psyche but on the entire nervous system."

In a recent study, the first in an emerging research area, Brian Bride of the University of Georgia found that exposure to others' trauma doubles the risk that social workers will experience posttraumatic stress disorder. He found numerous indicators of secondary trauma and illuminated the fact that while the rate of secondary trauma among social workers is high, their awareness of trauma's effects on them is low. "Social workers may hear about burnout, and they may hear about self-care," Bride says, "but they're not hearing about secondary post-traumatic stress disorder."

When we focus on our trauma exposure response, what exactly does it look like? What are the specifics? In the next chapter, we'll survey 16 common consequences of trauma exposure. These results often occur on a continuum: Some changes are very slight and may not even be noticed by you or your friends, while others may be dramatic and life changing. Different people will experience the consequences of trauma exposure in very different ways. Still, patterns do emerge, and they can help us to recognize and address our response.

While our feelings or behavior may be quite evident, it may nonetheless be difficult to identify trauma exposure as their cause. During an interview with American correspondent Ray Suarez on National Public Radio, Desmond Tutu, the South African archbishop and anti-apartheid activist, provided a striking example of how difficult it can be to stay present to our own responses even when our experience of trauma is indirect. He described a chilling scene that took place during South Africa's post-apartheid Truth and Reconciliation

Commission hearings. He was working closely with a woman whose job was to record the oral testimony. At one point, she looked down to see her hands drenched with her tears. She had no knowledge of her own weeping, even as she continued typing the detailed testimonies.

Just like that stenographer, many of us develop coping mechanisms that serve us extremely well—in the moment. Outside the moment of crisis, they may no longer provide any benefit. And yet, even with the passage of time, the changing of circumstances, and our own individual growth, we continue to employ our now-outdated coping skills. They are familiar to us, and we are experts at using them. We may even have inherited some of them from generations before us. But eventually they may reach a point where they are not just ineffective—they imprison us.

For many of us, the elaborate architecture we build around our hearts begins to resemble a fortress. We build up our defenses, but the trauma keeps on coming. We add a moat, we throw in some crocodiles, we forge more weapons, we build higher and higher walls. Sooner or later, we find ourselves locked in by the very defenses we have constructed for our own protection. We will find the key to our liberation only when we accept that what we once did to survive is now destroying us. And thus we begin the work of dismantling our fortress, releasing the crocodiles back to their habitat, and melting down the weapons to recycle into plowshares. Rather than fend off life, we slowly train ourselves to open our hearts to everything that comes to the door.

In his book *Waking the Tiger,* Peter Levine, a pioneering researcher and psychologist in the trauma field and founder of the concept of somatic experiencing, writes, "Today, our survival depends increasingly on developing our ability to think rather than being able to physically respond. Consequently, most of us have become separated from our natural, instinctual selves—in particular, the part of us that can proudly, not disparagingly, be called animal.... The fundamental challenges we face today have come about relatively quickly, but our nervous systems have been much slower to change. It is no coincidence that people who are more in touch with their natural selves tend to fare better when it comes to trauma."

As Levine suggests, we are often rewarded when we deny or displace our feelings. It is critical to remember that while aspects of our trauma exposure response may have served us in some capacity or may continue to serve us in some capacity, and may be socially and institutionally supported, we are exploring them from the standpoint of "How is this working for my deepest, most honest self? How is this working for those I serve? How is this sustainable? What is a more functional way to respond?"

Acknowledging a trauma exposure response can be difficult for any number of reasons. Many caregivers feel guilty for struggling with their work because, they tell themselves, who are they to complain about their lives? A conservation biologist working in Sierra Leone told me, "I never wanted to give my afflictions any credibility by acknowledging their impact on my life, as that would distract and detract from those who truly suffered." Others may be convinced that they should be able to rise above all this and that feelings of distress are a sign of weakness.

Secretly, many of us may feel that if we admit to having a hard time, we will open a door that we won't know how to shut. In organizations where toughness is promoted as a virtue, there may be a great deal of incentive to keep up our façade. As one community organizer told me, "I think we're all fronting with how we're doing."

Being open to the existence of our trauma exposure response is a critical step in trauma stewardship. I have no attachment to convincing you, the reader, that you are suffering from such exposure. I'm just encouraging you to explore the possibility of unexpected consequences from your work. Openness is critical. "There's liberation in reality," as the American jazz saxophonist Branford Marsalis has said.

By coming into the present moment again and again, we can gain crucial awareness of our trauma exposure response and, further, what would be helpful to us. The healing process may require a continuous effort to realize and re-realize that our trauma exposure response is not going away unless we give it proper attention. The sooner the better for this realization, since we are hoping to consider this from a preventive standpoint when possible, because, as those who are savvy in the ways of the human body will tell you, "by the time you're thirsty, you're already dehydrated." Cultivating awareness will allow us to gauge our thirst level and assess what we need to do about it. If we can recognize any of these shifts early, we can often limit their negative impact on our lives. Ignoring the red flags of a trauma exposure response is akin to ignoring the early rumblings of an avalanche or dismissing the signs for a dangerous cliff up ahead on the trail.

When I was a social worker in the trauma center at Harborview Medical Center in Seattle, the Level 1 trauma center for the Pacific Northwest, I marveled at how some of the doctors could distance themselves from their feelings. When someone died, a doctor and a social worker went into a small room called "the quiet room" and the doctor conveyed the news to the patient's loved ones. He or she would answer any questions and then leave, and the social worker would remain with the family.

I remember feeling like I was in an altered reality as I saw the distant look in the doctors' eyes and heard the hollowness in their voices as they talked with families. While these things were deeply unsettling, I fully understood that if I had to choose between that doctor saving the life of someone I loved and that doctor being a compassionate, active listener, I'd choose the former. I knew that doctors and nurses trying desperately to help critically injured patients had to develop an immediate way of coping. And yet it was evident that this compartmentalizing and numbing was not wholly sustainable. There was a personal and professional cost, both to the providers and to those around them.

Of course, people respond to trauma exposure in many ways that are not included in this book, but I have included the most common experiences in chapter 4. Again, a reminder: remain curious, take deep breaths, and maintain a sense of humor as you consider how this information applies to you. Only by understanding the topography of the land that you are lost in can you begin to plot the wisest way out.

CHAPTER FOUR

The 16 Warning Signs of Trauma Exposure Response

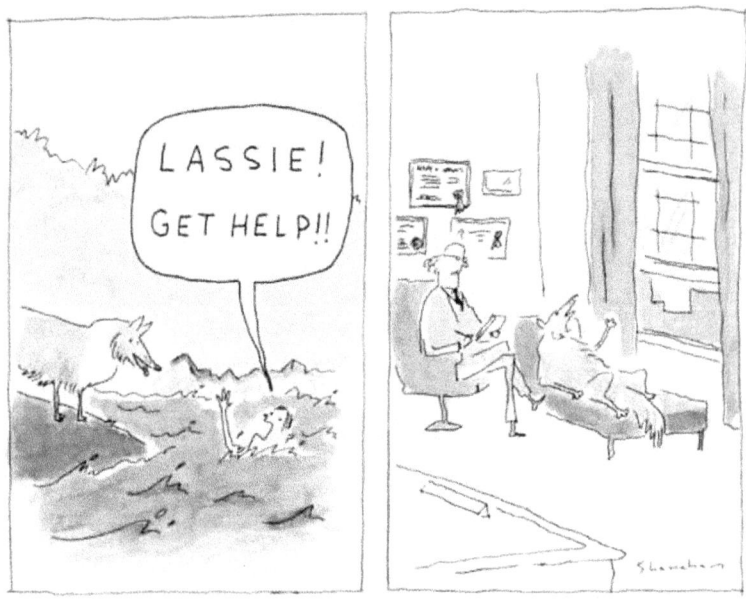

Figure 4.1

As you make your way through the 16 signs of trauma exposure response, take note of how you feel. For some people I work with, the experience of analyzing their trauma exposure response can be quite unsettling. Recently, at a statewide cervical cancer conference where we were reviewing trauma exposure response, a participant leaned over to her colleague and said, "I swear she must have talked to my partner." Her colleague responded, "Well, then she gets around, because she most certainly has talked to mine as well!" Some feel as if there's an intervention being planned and they alone are at the center of it. Some worry that there is something wrong with them. Still others become immediately overwhelmed. I remind them, and I would like to remind my readers, that whether you identify with many of the warning signs, a few, or none at all, you are more than okay. It is perfectly normal to have a response to trauma exposure. This means you still have the capacity to connect your internal world with the external reality, and this, as you know, is a great blessing. As hard as it is to feel our full range of feelings, still more damaging are our attempts to not feel. Even if we don't believe we have any trauma exposure response, what compassion and insight can we bring to those who do? As we move ahead, we can honor ourselves for having the courage to look honestly at our own behavior. Already, we have taken the first step toward more effective trauma stewardship.

Feeling Helpless and Hopeless

> I have witnessed mass mortality of frogs in Panama, and we can now predict this disease's path, and to some degree its date of arrival. We can't do anything to stop it, or help the frogs in the wild. It is so incredibly unusual and unbelievable, and sad. We all believe we will continue to lose a lot more amphibian species before we get anywhere close to solving this.
> Karen Lips, associate professor, University of Maryland Department of Biology

A person experiencing hopelessness or helplessness may wake up in the morning with that "Why am I even getting out of bed?" feeling. It may be hard to see that any progress is being made for positive social or environmental change. Victor Pantesco, a pioneering researcher of trauma's impact on conservationists and biologists, says this is often true for those who work in the field. "We're talking about people who are on the daily front lines of the planet, and they see the planet being affected in catastrophic ways, with a speed that crosses a threshold of manageability. They don't have an escape. It all just gets too big." Even though a person may be part of a very successful program, environmental or otherwise, the positive may be eclipsed and the negative exalted. Successes, markers of improvement, and the opportunities for growth can be hard to keep in focus. Instead, a person may believe only that things are plunging into greater despair and chaos—locally, nationally, and worldwide. Personally, one may feel overwhelmed, as if nothing can remedy the situation. I lived in Guatemala, where the ravages of the war were still very present in people's lives. They frequently used the expression *No vale la pena,* which translates to "It's not worth the pain." That made a strong impression on me. I imagined that the expression had been born out of the prolonged sufferings of war and poverty, and that the people had an increased sense of what was worth the effort and what was not. It was as if they were already down to their last reserves of energy and hopefulness, and they weren't about to threaten their precious remaining resources by engaging with pain that might drain them still further. (Figure 4.2)

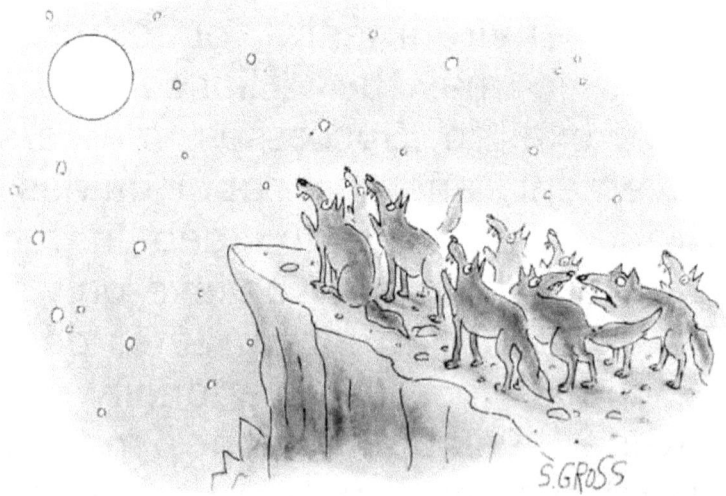

Figure 4.2: "My question is: Are we making an impact?"

Kirsten Stade, an environmental scientist who also takes in foster dogs and cats, told me about her struggles with feelings of helplessness. "With the environmental work, I often succumb to a feeling of impotence, that any issue I work on, any awareness I raise, is just such an insignificant drop in the massive bucket of impending crisis. The work I do with animals brings its own unique challenges. On the one hand, this work is enormously rewarding because every act of animal rescue has an immediate, tangible result: One life has been saved. The struggle comes from the knowledge, again, that whatever I do is pitiably inadequate to the task. So though every act of rescuing brings the knowledge of a life saved, it also brings the knowledge of countless lives not saved. This to me feels like personal failure."

A Ph.D. candidate in ecology described another aspect of feeling hopeless and helpless. She began her work in the Peruvian Amazon in 1996, as a 21-year-old undergraduate, and continued it through graduate school. She said,

I grew up in northern Michigan and spent most of my free time playing in the woods and lakes but, also, as the daughter of journalists, was immersed in world news. I was incredibly idealistic and wanted to help make a difference. In Peru, the elders asked me to study and document community-based fisheries management. The national government views the community's efforts as illegal, while the people view local management as both a right and an immediate necessity to ensure that the resources upon which they depend continue into the future. They hoped that documenting some of the practices might help change national policy.

It was incredibly fulfilling work, but also very lonely and harrowing at times. Despite community efforts, the fishery had clearly begun to collapse, and in 1999 high floods led to actual starvation.

When I came home, I was severely depressed and diagnosed with vicarious traumatization. I told people that I felt like I had been banging my head against a brick wall and the only dents that had been made were in my now very bloody skull. The hardest thing for me, in general, is that I feel overwhelmed by the level of need, the lack of empowerment, and the fact that nothing I do seems to make a difference. I often end up wondering why I didn't study to be a doctor. I know that to some extent I am coping by not letting myself fully look things in the face at the moment, and I want to find a better path.

In the course of extensive research, Judy Garber and Martin E.P. Seligman identified three types of perceptions that contribute directly to feelings of helplessness among people in traumatic circumstances. First, individuals hold themselves personally responsible for a troubled situation even when no one could reasonably be expected to master it. Many workers can relate to this feeling: You know in your gut that there is only so much you can do, but you still feel responsible in some way. Second, individuals perceive that the traumatic event itself will be long-lived—they see no possibility of relief. This applies particularly to workers who view their work as their career and not a time-limited job. Unyielding focus on a single field may leave workers feeling in over their heads and unable to see even a glimmer of light at the end of the tunnel. Third, individuals believe that they are likely to repeat their current struggles in another time and place. Workers who feel they are not functioning well in a specific trauma-related situation may imagine that they will experience the same difficulties in all similar situations. A person with such an attitude is likely to experience a greater sense of helplessness than someone who understands each situation to be a specific instance and not an indicator of future coping capacity.

A conversation I heard between two women who are friends and colleagues in post-Katrina New Orleans illustrates how overwhelming these feelings can be:

"I want to go home, but I don't have a home to go home to—my daughters aren't there, my neighbors aren't there, my doctor's not there."

"I know it's hard, but everything passes in time. You know, in 10 years this won't seem so bad. I know that seems like a long time, but..."

"Yeah, that does feel like a long time. Right now, one day feels like a long time."

PROFILE VANCE VREDENBURG

SAN FRANCISCO, CALIFORNIA
CURRENTLY: Assistant professor in the Department of Biology at San Francisco State University; cofounder and assistant director of AmphibiaWeb, an amphibian bioinformatics and conservation organization; research associate at the University of California, Berkeley's Museum of Vertebrate Zoology and at the California Academy of Sciences.

FORMERLY: Postdoctoral scholar, Department of Integrative Biology and Museum of Vertebrate Zoology, University of California, Berkeley.

I am an ecologist. My area of study is amphibian ecology, conservation, and evolution. I actually got started working in marine science, mostly fishes but also crustaceans, and I was once even hired as an algae specialist. My work over the past 20 years has taken me from Alaska to Antarctica, from the Caribbean to Guatemala and Mexico, and even as far as Asia. Although my passion now is studying amphibians, I began investigating them as an ecologist. I wasn't one of those kids who were chasing frogs from age four.

As an undergrad and for five years after, I studied sexual selection in marine fishes. When it came to graduate school, I looked for a project with more of a conservation angle. I wanted my scientific work to feed back directly to preserve this beautiful world we live in. I was lucky to find a project in the Sierra Nevada—in California. It's an amazing place to work. These natural parks and wilderness areas are some of our planet's most protected habitats, but it turns out that amphibians—frogs, toads, salamanders—have been disappearing even here. In the Sierra Nevada, we're talking about frogs who live in areas with no roads for hundreds of miles and who move maybe only a few hundred meters in their entire lives. So why are we losing them?

I came in as a conservation biologist at the time knowing little about amphibians. But when I began to study mountain yellow-legged frogs [a species listed as critically endangered], I tested an idea that others had totally brushed aside. I wanted to further explore this idea that the introduction of species was causing the decline of these frogs. People introduced trout into areas that historically had no fish, and the trout ate the frogs, but no one was there to watch it happen. I basically did classic ecological experiments to show that the introduction of nonnative trout has decimated frog populations in these supposedly pristine areas. The truth is that even our most protected areas have been greatly changed, sometimes in subtle ways, by humans. My research was really exciting, because in this time of worldwide amphibian decline there are next to no examples of frogs recovering after declines. In this case, I found that if you restored the habitat to its natural condition, the frogs rebounded and quickly, so imagine this ray of hope! It was just incredible.

The Park Service and other federal and state agencies quickly realized that this was a simple and elegant way to turn around these amphibian declines. They took my Ph.D. thesis and turned it into actual conservation action. Think about how meaningful this could be for these frogs—a graduate student's efforts scaled up to the level of federal and state agencies with many more resources to bring to the situation. Exactly what I was hoping to do with my life! And then just as the frogs were starting to recover, just as the conservation actions were implemented on a much larger landscape and things were turning around—just then I started finding first dozens and then tens of thousands of dead frogs. You can imagine what the effect was on me personally. After seven years of monitoring populations, conducting experiments, publishing papers, and proving to people that something could be done to help these amphibians, my colleagues and I started finding dead frogs. It turned out it was an emerging disease.

The impact was devastating. We had put in all that hard work. I could see a future where these amphibians could be restored to their original state and saved from extinction. Having the whole ecosystem revert to a more natural state was good not only for the frogs but for all the species in the food web. The interconnected web of life was suddenly moving back in the right direction—the algae, the plants, the frogs, the coyotes, the raven, the bears. And now all that was unraveling.

I was overtaken by a sense of doom that there really is nothing we can do to reverse this worldwide decline of species. I'd heard about this disease affecting amphibians in other places. I had thought, "It's not gonna happen here," but it did. It just destroyed me. There was this beautiful alpine lake that was home to populations I'd sat with for years while they were being restored. I remember sitting on the shoreline just crying my heart out amidst hundreds of dead frogs. I had gone from this positive position of feeling that we had the power to turn things around to realizing that I was absolutely powerless. I had been working on this single project for nine years, and suddenly entire populations went extinct in a matter of months. Looking out over that quiet landscape, I thought, "There may be a time not far away when they are all extinct, and there's nothing I can do about it." I felt like I wanted to jump off a cliff or something, because the spirit had just dropped out of me. I had an emotional connection to these really beautiful animals that I personally had helped by giving their habitat back. I had seen this vibrant life return to this area and now I was seeing it all disappear and I couldn't do anything. I can't really describe the feeling—it was like floating back down to earth. I went from, wow, humans can do these great things and people are lining up to help to ... nada, worthless. That was really, really, really hard.

So what in the world is going on with this disease? I finally picked myself up and found a bunch of smart people to write a proposal with, and we got funded by the National Science Foundation to go and find out why this is causing such massive mortality. It's the worst case in recorded history of a disease driving species to extinction. And it jumps between species of amphibians. Some might ask, "Who cares?" Well, I care because I care about amphibians, but everyone should care. Think about it: If this type of deadly disease got into a human population or into the organisms that we depend on for our survival (corn, rice, wheat, cattle, poultry), it would be catastrophic. There is very good reason to keenly understand a disease like this. Why is it killing amphibians, how is it spreading, is there a way to slow down the effects? There are a lot of big questions that are very interesting purely for science but also for conservation and for our general understanding of emerging diseases. Hundreds of species of amphibians have gone extinct because of this disease. The one hopeful thing we've found is that some species are surviving, so we're looking at the coexistence between the deadly fungus and those species. We still don't have any solid answers, but we do know more than we did four or five years ago.

I have traveled to Mexico and Guatemala and am working with colleagues in Sri Lanka, Madagascar, the Philippines, Thailand, Laos, and China to see if it's killing species and where. Back in the Sierra Nevada I'm trying out techniques to slow down the effects of the disease and to help the frogs survive the epidemic. Two years ago I got permission from the National Park Service to go treat some frogs in an epidemic using an antifungal bath. So far, it looks like it worked. I'm trying to convince the Park Service to try this on a bigger scale with more populations that lie in the path of this disease. Several researchers are also working with zoos to try to get in front of these waves of mortality and save some of these species before they go extinct. We are bringing a few individuals into captivity to keep them safe. We're trying to get them to breed so that some day we can reintroduce them to the wild, but this is uncharted territory and no one knows if it will be successful. This is unbelievable, how much destruction this disease has caused. It's like nothing we've ever seen before.

I'm linking up with researchers all around the world to look at this problem. When calamities happen, folks all over the planet come together. That's what's going on in the scientific community. It's such a dramatic and dangerous thing that rivalries have gone away and people are coming together and sharing information and trying to figure out what we can do.

I just coauthored a paper with David Wake that has gotten a lot of press because it concludes that the amphibians are signaling that we are entering the sixth mass extinction of life on Earth. In the history of life on Earth there have been five mass extinctions, or periods of time where life on Earth nearly went extinct. The most drastic one, the Permian-Triassic Extinction, occurred 250 million years ago, and 95 percent of life on Earth went extinct. By the way, amphibians survived that one! We think that right now we're entering another phase of mass extinction, and the amphibians are the sentinels. They are telling us that something is wrong. More than a third of the world's 6,300 amphibian species are threatened with extinction.

It's disheartening, to say the least. Good god, what's going to happen? We have one earth, and there's nowhere else to live. People tend to forget that. It's difficult to look at bad news, but you can't put this aside. In my job I'm confronted with it on a daily basis. I'm studying this group of organisms that has been around for 300 million years, and right now as I'm watching them, in my short life, they're going extinct.

Sometimes I'd like to go work on something happy, like a children's film for Pixar, but instead I work on gloom and doom. I got into this because I love nature and I care about our world. I feel absolutely privileged to be in these beautiful places with these gorgeous animals, but watching them struggle and die in my hands is the saddest thing I've ever seen. I've always had this idea that if I ever had children, I'd take them up and show them these amazing frogs. Now what am I going to do? Is there going to be any place left or are they just going to see it on a computer screen?

And that is a horrible thought. I see so much beauty in life, but when I see species disappearing, I wonder what is going to be left. I don't want to be Mr. Grim, but that's what I'm confronted with. Sometimes I just get really sad. Science is about facts, and there's no avoiding the truth.

The conservation side of our field has grown by leaps and bounds, and we are all trying to study different angles of this problem. People have come together and collaborated in a way no one did in the past. There's also this impending doom. The older generation of scientists talk about places all over the world that used to be full of amphibians, and they talk about all the wonderful night hikes they'd go on and you go there now and there's nothing there. At many sites, over 40 percent of the species are gone forever. In Costa Rica, at the Monteverde Cloud Forest Reserve, there used to be over 20 species of amphibians. Today you are lucky if you see one. I feel robbed on some level. If something is extinct, there's nothing you can do about it. There are plenty of stories from older scientists that talk about what they'd seen and how abundant this salamander or that frog was, and you go out at night these days and it's completely silent because there's not a single amphibian calling.

Scientists aren't supposed to feel very much. We like talking about data and facts and hypotheses. We don't usually talk about feelings, especially not when we're in a crowd, but with this topic you hear the sadness and despair come through. It creeps out during scientific talks. There's a silence in the room and you can feel it. Before this doom and gloom came, people at meetings would get together and talk about new findings. Now there's a lot of talk about what has been lost and what is going to be hit next and what can be done. The tone has changed from excitement and discovery to bewilderment and sadness.

It's really hard to be enthusiastic about getting other people to study amphibians when I know that eventually they'll hit this sad truth. I hope I don't lose it so badly that I don't want to encourage people to get excited about science and research and nature, but it's pretty hard. When grad students ask to work in my lab, I think, "Are they going to be able to deal with the animals dying?" I never thought about that before. I used to feel much more hope that we could turn things around. Now, with things happening at the worldwide level, I think some of the problems are insurmountable. That's a big, big change for me. I try to stay positive and focused on the few cases where we might make a difference. I think we're poised to turn things around in the U.S., at least culturally. We can use education to teach people to keep biodiversity in mind. That is very important to us changing things.

    I don't know that there's a good way to find peace with this. Realizing that bad things happen is an understanding that is part of life, but I always thought that bad things could be turned around. With extinction there's nothing left to fix. There may be a fundamental lesson about hopelessness, but I had never let it sink in.

I try to tell myself that even though I haven't seen it, there must be something we can do. Maybe there's a way we won't lose everything. I tell myself, let me quickly learn what I can right now. The whole scientific community feels this way. It's such a crisis that the scientific community is willing to do things now that we wouldn't have been willing to do 10 years ago. We're now trying riskier things. Science is becoming more flexible. A few years ago, we thought if we couldn't get a research paper out of it, we were wasting our time. Now we're like, "Screw it, we'll do it anyway." We need the agencies that fund science to allow more flexibility.

I feel a sense of pressure that goes well beyond having to turn in my next report, to get a manuscript published, or to get this research done. The pressure is phenomenal. I had no idea how much pressure there is. I feel like I need 10 copies of myself to keep up, and it's not even close to being enough. Extinction is really forever. I can't stress how much weight that puts on my life. Sometimes I wake up at three in the morning thinking about all I need to do to move this research forward. It's not for my career—that doesn't even matter. It's that feeling of despair and sense that we've got to do something! This is the last breath of air and you've got to do everything you can, or you're not going to make it back up to the surface. It's like this not just for me, but for everyone in my field. And you don't want to live life that way all the time.

A Sense That One Can Never Do Enough

It's not a feeling, it's true. If I don't do it, it's not going to get done, and if it doesn't get done, people die. I can never do enough. Attorney for inmates sentenced to capital punishment (Figure 4.3)

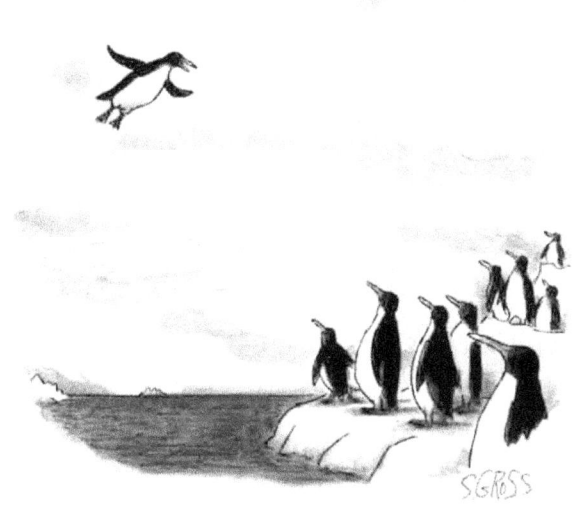

Figure 4.3: "We just haven't been flapping them hard enough."

The belief that "I am not doing enough and I should be doing more" is widespread and often a powerful influence on our lives. Often, this belief dates back to the early years of our lives. As children, what messages did we receive about sustainability and longevity? Did we get the word that "It's a long road—take good care of yourself, prioritize your health and your well-being"? Or did the repeated messages lead us to internalize the oppressive lesson that "No matter what you do or how you do it, it won't be enough"?

Nobody is immune from circumstances that instill a sense of inadequacy. Almost everyone has had to withstand negative teachings to some degree. At the same time, certain people are likely to receive these lessons more often and in more ways than others. Many of us are members of one or more social groups for which the oppressive messages are continually reinforced.

We can view this notion of scarcity and "not enough-ness" from a larger framework of systematic oppression. Oppression is most commonly felt and expressed as a widespread, if unconscious, belief that a certain group of people are inferior. We often attribute such bias to individuals. But when such feelings as racism, sexism, homophobia, and classism are codified into law or integrated into the functioning of social systems, this becomes systematic oppression.

The most obvious forms of oppression typically begin with the denigration and dehumanization of certain individuals or groups. This may escalate to scapegoating, which may in turn lead to aggression against the targeted parties that can take many forms—from individual violence to government legislation. When the victims of oppression come to believe the misinformation used to denigrate or dehumanize them, the result is "internalized oppression." Ultimately, internalized oppression can drive members of targeted groups to turn the methods of the oppressor on each other or themselves. For example, female case managers may internalize social messages that women should be compliant, cooperative, and grateful. So, while men who contact human service agencies with an assertive sense of entitlement to effective services may be met with deference, women who present with the same tone may be dismissed as undeserving, combative, litigious, or "borderline"—especially in fields predominantly staffed by female workers.

A particularly powerful component of internalized oppression arises when its victims come to believe in a notion of scarcity. The oppressor creates a climate in which people fear there is not enough room for everyone, and so they begin a desperate attempt to conform to the oppressor's ideals in order to survive. This can happen on an individual, group, community, or even societal level. People accept the negative stereotypes that say they are not good enough, and they begin to strive, largely unconsciously, toward a rigid idea of what may be acceptable. They may also attempt to impose their externally derived standards of right and wrong on other members of their communities, often quite harshly. Within targeted communities, this dynamic can contribute to pervasive and brutal strife. On an individual level, it creates people who are never able to feel that who they are is enough. These people may seek protection by striving for the trappings of an idealized life in which they might someday measure up as "enough." This looks different for everyone throughout the world, and yet at the risk of overgeneralizing, we can see some persistent themes. (Figure 4.4)

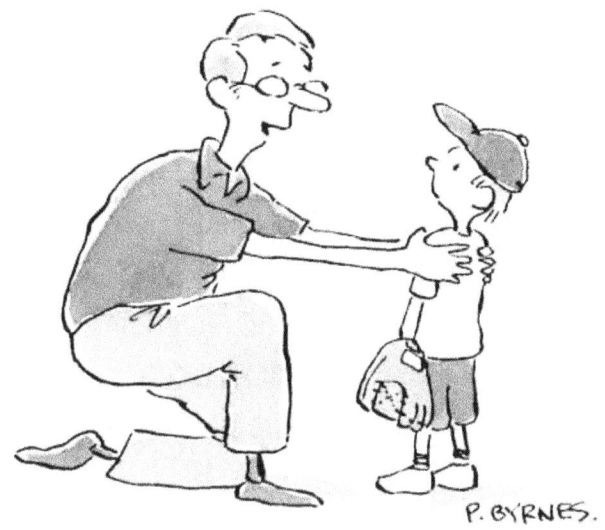

Figure 4.4: "Just remember, son, it doesn't mailer whether you win or lose—unless yon want Daddy's love."

I know from my membership and experience in Black communities that there is a widely held belief that if we work hard enough, if we labor long enough, if we produce enough, then we'll be safe. In Jewish communities, I've experienced this as an emphasis on learning: If we're learned enough, if we are intellectual enough, if we are in our heads enough, then we'll avoid suffering. Being born and raised female,

I internalized messages that taught me that if I nurture others enough, if I care enough, if I anticipate others' needs enough, then everything will be okay. We can look at the groups we belong to and remember the messages we received from those who raised us, and from our society, and assess what we've come to believe about ourselves. Will we ever be "Black enough" or "man enough" or "gay enough"? The larger oppression model argues that this line of socialization leads to further oppression within and between groups, and leaves individuals with a deep, lingering sense of not being enough ... ever. (Figure 4.5)

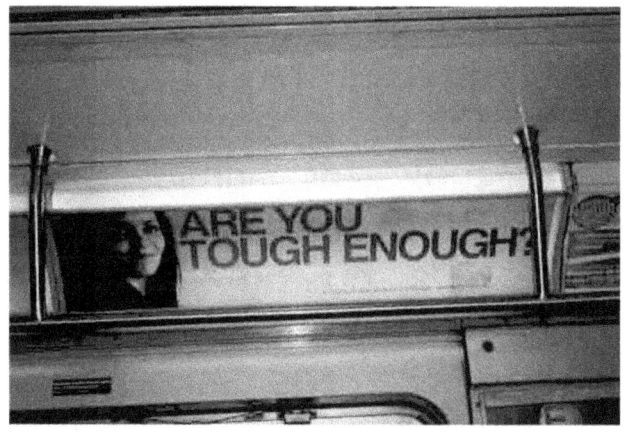
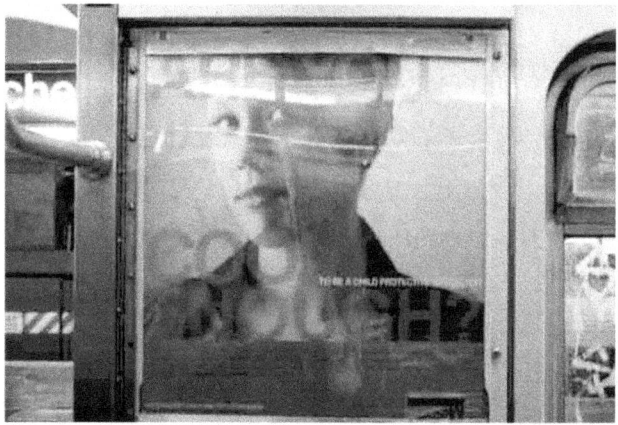
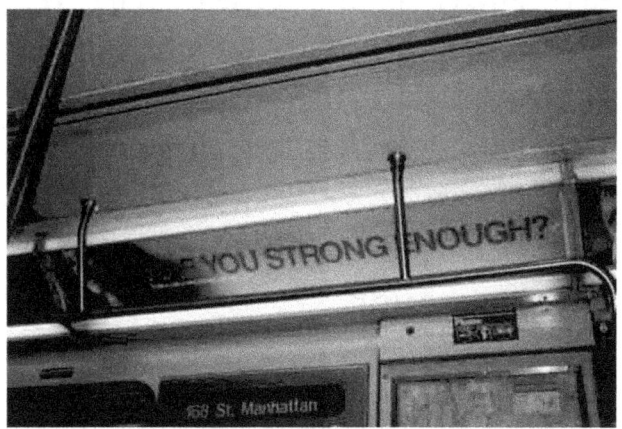

Figure 4.5: Yuko Uchikawa

New York City's Administration for Children's Services (ACS) has actually used a challenge to be "enough" as a recruiting tool for child protective specialists. The agency created a series of subway ads posing questions that were intended to recruit potential hires. One by one, the ads asked, "Are you clear enough?" "Are you brave enough?" "Are you cool enough?" "Are you wise enough?" "Are you smart enough?" "Are you strong enough?" "Are you good enough?" "Are you bold enough?" "Are you tough enough?" "Are you calm enough?" "Are you kind enough?" "Are you real enough?"

While ACS's reasons for designing this campaign were based in a desire to deliver the best possible services to the families they serve, it is worth exploring the impact of such messages. We can consider how this ethos manifests in our fields of work. When I facilitate workshops on trauma stewardship, I rarely hear from participants that they work or volunteer in places that encourage them to take care of themselves, to pace themselves at a sustainable rate, or to maintain balance in their lives. Many of our fields and places of work seem to function, instead, from a place of tremendous urgency. This sense of urgency distracts many organizations from addressing how to best retain healthy, happy people who will continue to contribute to the betterment of the world. It's very common to see an internalization of not doing enough pervading our workplaces. When our personal belief that we are not enough collides with our professional belief that we're not doing enough, we can feel like we're coming apart at the seams. And the haunting questions—Am I good enough? Am I tough enough? Am I smart enough?—can confuse our ability to be honest about how we're actually doing, day to day. Every day that passes, we think to ourselves that we haven't done enough because we're not being enough. We're often left with limitless dissatisfaction in our work and lives.

As vice curator of the education department, part of my work was to attract more youngsters into the field of conservation. The more I worked, the more facts about conservation and animal welfare I had to know. This information made me feel sad and despairing, and I would get angry easier. Eventually, I left the job.

Now I still do my best to help animals, but I do not want to know more about the details of the animals' plight. Sometimes I feel guilty for bringing young people into this field, because I know this job is hard for their feelings and emotions. They probably will not be as happy as they used to be. Sorry, I know I am not a strong woman.

Luo Lan, conservation educator, People's Republic of China

Hypervigilance

I eat in a hurry—I do everything in a hurry because I feel like there is a ticking time bomb waiting to go off.

Community activist

I remember being 18 years old, working in a domestic violence shelter.

I watched the child residents and was awed by their awareness of everything that was going on around them—24 hours a day, seven days a week, 360 degrees. They knew the welfare system, the immigration system, the legal system. And they were seven years old. Recently I was working with a group of outreach workers for homeless youth and women in the sex trade, and one of them shared that she had a very hard time staying emotionally present in her relationships. "My husband often asks me where I am," she said. "Even when you're with him?" I asked. "Especially when I'm with him," she answered. "Even on our honeymoon."

    Hypervigilance in our work creates a dynamic of being wholly focused on our job, to the extent that being present for anything else in our life can seem impossible. It is often an attempt to restore safety and prevent any further victimization by anticipating and recognizing everything as a potential threat and acting accordingly.

    This experience is common for many people who have survived trauma. In 2006, Seattle's Jewish Federation experienced a hate crime when a man entered the building and shot several people. A survivor's husband described how after the shooting, the level of his alertness to his surroundings went through the roof. He couldn't see his environment in any sort of measured context. Everything felt exaggerated, significant, and dangerous to him. (Figure 4.6)

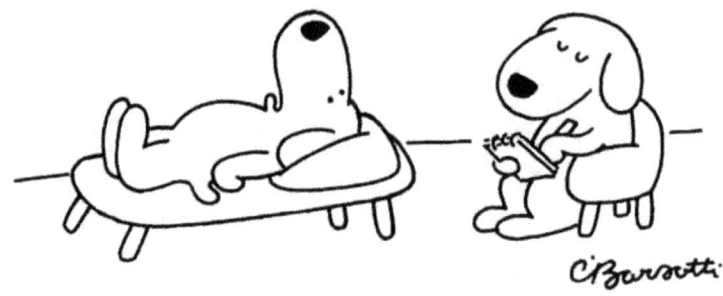

Figure 4.6: "I bark at everything. Can't go wrong that way"

I recently received photos from a friend's wedding, and as I sat there looking through them, I thought to myself, "I wonder when the domestic violence is going to start."

Domestic Violence Protection Order advocate

The same effect can happen over time with people who regularly bear witness to others' trauma. Having a trauma exposure response can make us feel like we're always "on," even during times when there is absolutely nothing that can or should be done. There is no rest for the weary. As one AmeriCorps worker who is based in a police department said, "I assess everything from a crime risk perspective—every building, every open place, every location."

Elaine Miller-Karas, educator, psychotherapist, and cofounder of the Trauma Resource Institute, has helped develop a model called Trauma First Aide. Trauma First Aide can be used in time-limited situations to stabilize the nervous systems of people who have had traumatic experiences. According to this model, the nervous system's natural swings between internal sensations of well-being (or comfort) and tension (or discomfort) get interrupted during overwhelming events. Some people get stuck in a state of hyperarousal, which can include hypervigilance and heightened states of anxiety; others may sink into states of numbness or depression. People may spend extended periods at either extreme, rather than returning to an ideal state of homeostasis or balance. Miller-Karas worked with first responders and survivors both in Thailand and on the Gulf Coast, and she recounts that many of them came to "live in states of dysregulation fluctuating between being stuck on 'high' or 'low.' If we can help them regulate their nervous systems in the aftermath of what they have been through, then they can get back in their body and walk through their life. If you're frozen or in a state of hyperarousal all the time, you don't have the attention you need to do the work of healing. When you are able to attend to and stabilize your body, then you can be more present in mind, body, and spirit."

This can get complicated. Reasonable people may begin to feel that they are constantly surrounded by potential dangers. If you work in violence prevention and you listen to pop music, you may recognize that the majority of "love" songs are about stalking, that most "horror" films have a domestic violence theme, and so on. I remember the first time I shopped for my daughter in the Gap's "girls" section instead of its "toddlers" section. The provocative nature of the clothing for four- and five-year-olds was enough to put me over the edge, but then I realized there was more to pay attention to: The loud music playing throughout the department was entirely about a boy trying to track down and find a girl and why wasn't she taking his calls and what would he do without her? When it became unbearable after a mere two minutes, I went to the cashier and asked if it'd be possible to change the track, to which she replied that the music came out of Gap headquarters in San Francisco, and I'd need to contact them.

Our tendencies toward hypervigilance may be further reinforced by modern technology. By being connected and constantly informed, they say, we can increase our safety and keep our families safe. So the expectation increases that we be reachable and "on." First came voice mail and pagers, then cell phones and e-mail, and now BlackBerrys, Treos, iPhones, and other on-demand devices. Hypervigilance makes it difficult to ever turn off the information, get away from work, and relax and be present in our lives. This is a trend that has far-reaching implications, even miles away from our jobs. Stephanie Levine, a massage therapist and public school volunteer in Seattle, described the start of a vacation: "Once I arrived, I felt like I had to do everything immediately. Go for a walk, read a book, take a nap ... I had to hurry up and relax." This phenomenon transports us out of the present moment and keeps us anticipating what's next. We have the option to turn the devices off, but our own behavior is harder to shift. (Figure 4.7)

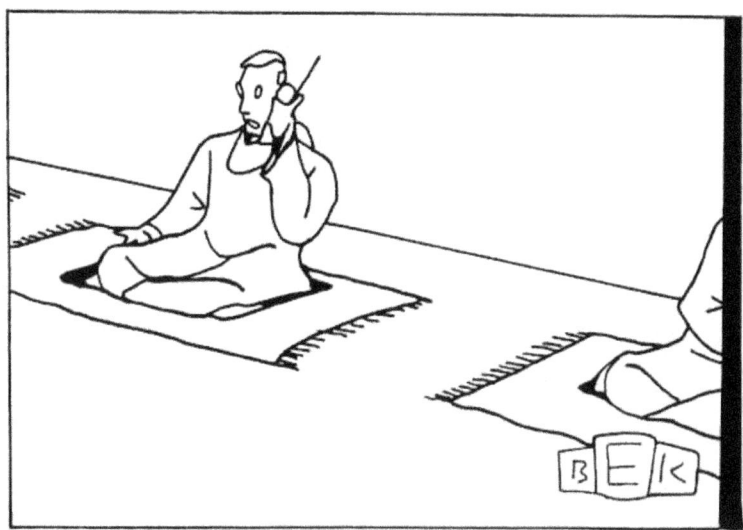

Figure 4.7: "I'm crazed with this noble path—let me get hack to you."

Diminished Creativity

> All my energy goes into just getting through my days. I don't meditate anymore or write; that's what I used to do at night. I don't do anything anymore but work and go home and watch TV.
>
> Community organizer

Diminished creativity is when you think to yourself, "When was the last time I had an original thought?" You may find that you're bored with what you're doing and you can't remember a time when you felt creative. This is a damaging state of mind, not only because our joy decreases, but also because we may be less innovative at work. Diminished creativity as a trauma exposure response may help explain the stagnant conditions in many of our fields of practice.

I often look around and think: Given all the brilliant, competent, tremendous people in so many fields, how is it that this is where we are in the 21st century? The goal of the founders of the domestic violence movement was not that, decades later, women and children would still be in shelters. The early leaders of the U.S. public school system could never have imagined the depth of the problems in our schools today. And how is it possible that in the midst of a global climate crisis, there has been such a dearth of creative solutions? One answer is this: The deeper we sink into a culture of trauma, the less flexible and original our thinking becomes.

> Alice laughed. "There is no use trying," she said: "one can't believe impossible things."

> "I daresay you haven't had much practice," said the Queen. "When I was your age, I always did it for half-an-hour a day. Why, sometimes I've believed as many as six impossible things before breakfast."
>
> Alice's Adventures in Wonderland and Through the Looking Glass
> Lewis Carroll, English author, logician, clergyman, and photographer

Creativity requires embracing a certain amount of chaos, and it demands some leaps of faith. The ancient Roman philosopher Cicero said, "Only the person who is relaxed can create, and to that mind, ideas flow like lightning." When we contend with trauma exposure, however, we often find ourselves craving more structure and less creativity. We may resist change even when existing structures are out of date and detrimental to us personally and professionally.

I had the privilege of working as an advocate with the Northwest Network of Bisexual, Trans, Lesbian and Gay

Survivors of Abuse. One thing we did to maintain some level of creativity was to substitute one staff meeting per month with a writing group that we had collectively formed. The staff size was small, and yet it was always hard to maintain the group; our built-in resistances kept us thinking that we should be doing more important things than writing down the latest theories and approaches to our work. Nevertheless, we remained committed. We knew that if we let day-to-day busywork consume all our time, we would not grow. And if we did not progress, the movement we were a part of would not move forward.

The practice of creativity among the Northwest Network staff continued to evolve over the years. From writing came new projects and community connections, and from those connections came new ways to frame and understand the work. The messiness of creativity and engagement made fertile ground for growth, change, and innovation. (Figure 4.8)

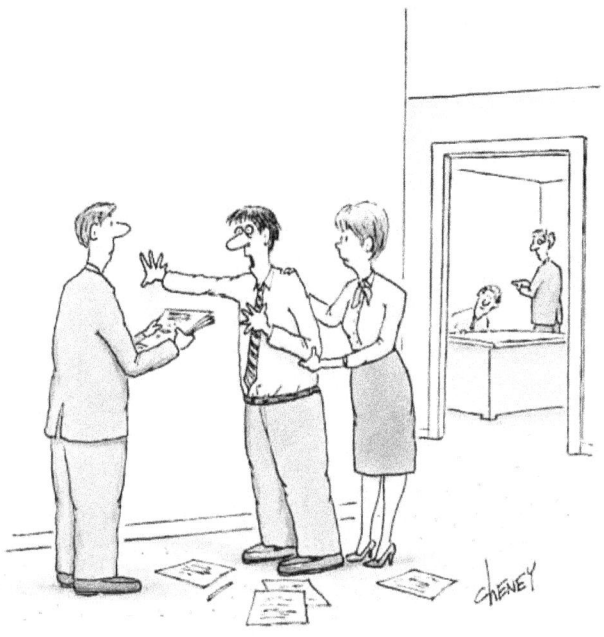

Figure 4.8: "Really, I'm fine. It was just a fleeting sense of purpose—I'm sure it will pass"

Over time, the Northwest Network's approach to its core work was transformed. Staff members challenged themselves to envision what they wanted to create in the world as clearly as they had previously defined what they wanted to end. While the organization originally understood its mission as "ending domestic violence," it came to understand that the greater work was to create the conditions necessary to support loving and equitable relationships.

The Northwest Network has grown from an agency offering first-rate traditional antiviolence services into a thriving and engaged community organization that is developing new and exciting strategies to end violence and create strong, loving communities.

Inability to Embrace Complexity

> There are more worlds than the one you can hold in your hand.
> Albert Hosteen, in The X-Files, "The Sixth Extinction II: Amor Fati," American science-fiction television series

There are strong indicators for the inability to embrace complexity: You crave clear signs of good and bad and right and wrong, and you feel an urgent need to choose sides. The answer "no" comes out of your mouth constantly, and you feel like your shoulders are up by your ears. Your explanations sound like bumper-sticker slogans and your thinking is fractured; there's no cohesive whole. You may be dogmatic and opinionated, and you may look to take a side in a debate no matter what the debate is about: All that concerns you is taking a stand. (Figure 4.9)

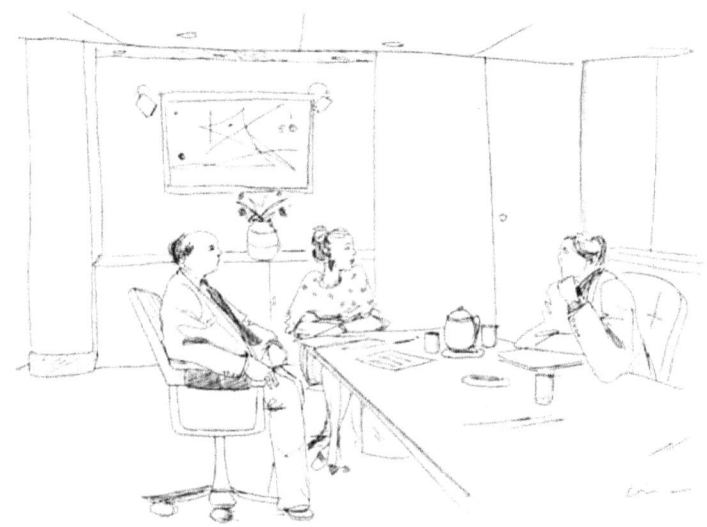

Figure 4.9: "What I'm proposing is this. No."

Taking sides can surface in workplace dynamics. We may see it in the form of gossip, cliques, divisions among staff, and rigid expectations of workers. As Billie Lawson, trauma social worker and foremother of the trauma exposure field, has said, "You cannot afford to negotiate roles when you're in the fray." You may feel like you're in high school, or worse yet, junior high. You don't hear positive statements like, "Wow, that program in south county seems to be having a hard time; I wonder how we can help them." Instead, it's much more negative and catty. You don't take a minute to check in with a colleague who seems to be struggling; it's more like, "I always knew she was going to be a train wreck." Taking sides can also show up in our clinical work, when we are unable to hold the entirety of a situation in our hands. Pay attention if you hear yourself making comments like "I love the mom I'm working with, but I really hate the dad."

This kind of behavior can have the same kinds of consequences as pouring fuel on a fire. No one steps in and says, "Let's slow down and think about this: What could be going on here? How else can we look at this? What have we forgotten to consider? What would be most helpful?" Instead, workers may escalate a volatile situation by making assumptions, passing judgment, talking about things they are not sure of, or engaging in any number of shortsighted behaviors.

Inability to manage complexity can show up in larger societal movements.

This was true of the domestic violence movement as it sought criminal penalties for people who batter, for instance. For what seemed like very good reasons at the time, its leaders limited the complexity of their response to domestic violence. Connie Burk explores this issue further in her account of the domestic violence movement's reliance on the criminal legal system, "A Question of Complexity".

> I learned to make my mind large, as the universe is large, so that there is room for paradoxes.
>
> Maxine Hong Kingston, Chinese-American writer, author of The Woman Warrior, and National Humanities Medal honoree

The inability to embrace complexity may be familiar to you if you have ever experienced primary trauma. Your individual need for the concrete elements of reality becomes paramount. Making room within yourself for all the complexities and gray areas is too painful and seems cognitively impossible. When we're rested, in a good space emotionally, and on our "A" game, we know that the world is a complex place; we know that seeing things through a flattened and reductionist lens does not serve us. And yet we live in a polarized civic universe: Our legal system is adversarial, as is our two-party-based political structure. We have zero-sum power systems embedded throughout our public institutions. You can only vote for or against. You can only be found guilty or not guilty. You can work for an initiative, work against an initiative, or be completely apathetic. And in the recent era of American politics, you're "either with me or you're with the terrorists."

What we see happening, then, is an internalization of binary structures that may at times work for large-scale governance but are almost never effective in the causes, predicaments, and relationships of everyday life. Most situations cry out for people to honor and understand the complexities of the situation.

This is challenging to put into practice. Embracing complexity doesn't mean that we should abandon the critique of cultural and social institutions that is so essential to social and environmental change work, nor does it mean that we should become complete moral relativists. We have an obligation to call out environmental racism, date rape, abuse within the prison industrial complex, and so on. And yet we misuse this responsibility to prophetic critique if we objectify and simplify what is happening.

I received a copy of a letter written by the Vietnamese Zen Buddhist monk and peace activist Thich Nhat Hanh to George Bush, then the president of the United States. In 1967, Thich Nhat Hanh was nominated for a Nobel Peace Prize by Martin Luther King Jr. for his efforts to end the Vietnam War. His life and work have provided a shining example of how we can continue to seek common ground, even with those who have ravaged our lives with violence. This letter is a powerful example of an attempt to change a situation while understanding its complex nature.

Dear Mr. President,

Last night i saw my brother (who died two weeks ago in the U.S.A.) coming back to me in a dream. He was with all his children. He told me, "Let's go home together." After a millisecond of hesitation, i told him joyfully, "OK, let's go."

Waking up from that dream at 5 am this morning, i thought of the situation in the Middle East; and for the first time, i was able to cry. I cried for a long time, and i felt much better after about one hour. Then i went in the kitchen and made some tea. While making tea, i realized that what my brother had said is true: our home is large enough for all of us. Let us go home as brothers and sisters.

Mr President, i think that if you could allow yourself to cry like i did this morning, you will also feel much better. It is our brothers that we kill over there. They are our brothers, God tells us so, and we also know it. They may not see us as brothers because of their anger, their misunderstanding, their discrimination. But with some awakening, we can see things in a different way, and this will allow us to respond differently to the situation. I trust God in you, i trust the Buddha nature in you. Thank you for reading.

In gratitude and with brotherhood
Thich Nhat Hanh
Plum Village (Figure 4.10)

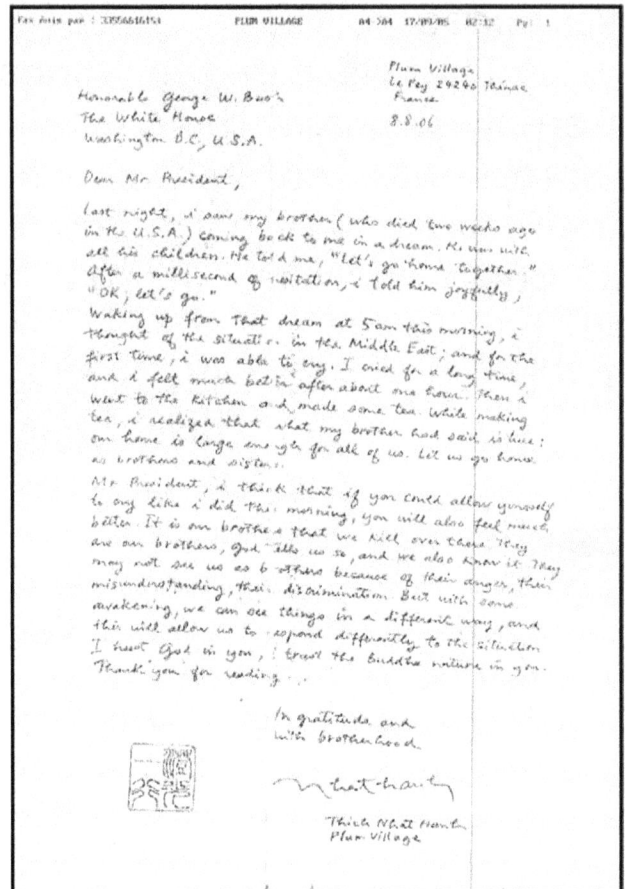

Figure 4.10: Letter courtesy of the Deer Park Monastery Web site

A QUESTION OF COMPLEXITY

Criminalization and the Movement to End Domestic Violence

When U.S. second-wave feminists began organizing against domestic violence in the late 1960s and 1970s, it was still legal in most states for a man to rape his wife, and only a handful of states had serious criminal consequences for wife battering. Husbands and lovers beat their partners with impunity—secure in the knowledge that the consequences, when there were any, would be manageable. The pain and suffering experienced by women beaten by their partners was minimized and denied. Women were told to be better wives. Men were told to take a walk around the block and cool off.

Advocates dedicated themselves to ending violence, and they knew that women's experiences of abuse would have to be taken seriously in order to make change. In U.S. courts, criminal offenses are viewed as harms not only to the victim but also to the entire society—that's why criminal cases are filed as *The State v. John Doe,* not *Jane Doe v. John Doe.* Women in the antiviolence movement believed that domestic violence and sexual assault would have to be acknowledged by the state as harms against society that should carry severe criminal consequences before any real change could happen.

Despite vocal misgivings from many in the field, the domestic violence movement oriented itself toward a criminal legal response. The urgency of the approach was repeatedly reinforced as women fleeing to domestic violence shelters shared horrific stories of violence at the hands of their husbands and partners, and conveyed devastating experiences of being dismissed or ignored by law enforcement and the courts when they tried to reach out for help. Some of the initial community-based responses to battering were abandoned as the apparent need for a criminal response began to eclipse other perspectives. In the years that followed, the movement brought the full force of its political and organizational will to bear on creating and sustaining a criminal legal response to domestic violence as the primary antiviolence strategy.

Thirty years later, in an enduring testament to the courage and dedication of its organizers, the movement had made great strides toward achieving its goals: Public awareness of the issue had skyrocketed, replacing a lethal history of silence about family violence with one of growing openness. Spousal rape is illegal in all 50 states, every state has felony domestic battery crimes, and most states have criminal courts dedicated to family violence. Issues of policing in response to domestic violence have been on the national agenda for over a decade. Meanwhile, even as the apparent victories mounted, another story was playing out across the nation. The United States increased its prison population from 300,000 in 1977 to over 2 million in 2005 (U.S. Department of Justice [DOJ], Bureau of Statistics). The number of people under correctional supervision (parole, probation, jail, prison) was over 7 million in 2005—up from fewer than 2 million in 1980. According to the U.S. DOJ, at year-end 2005, there were 3,145 Black male prison inmates per 100,000 Black males in the United States, compared with 1,244 Hispanic male inmates per 100,000 Hispanic males, and 471 white male inmates per 100,000 white males. Prison rape, HIV infection among incarcerated people, and other prison violence have escalated to a national crisis.

As the prison boom continued, efforts originally intended to protect people from violence and oppression became increasingly enmeshed with the criminal justice system. Shelter programs began to cooperate more and more with law enforcement and prosecutors. Some survivors who were reluctant to participate in prosecution came under greater scrutiny and pressure. In the past 10 years, domestic violence survivors have increasingly faced arrest and prosecution as a result of policing practices and battery laws that inadequately understand the experience of domestic violence. People of color, immigrants, and gay, lesbian, bisexual, and trans people have expressed their fears about the danger of overreliance on the criminal legal system. People in these communities have long been the targets of biased policing and harsh criminal prosecution or deportation.

For many in the domestic violence field, the concerns of survivors and marginalized communities came as a surprise. "How could criminalizing domestic violence possibly have negative consequences?" they asked. The majority of advocates were still fighting tirelessly for the vicious assaults against women to be taken seriously as a crime. To most of them, the virtues of the strategy were self-evident. Criminal penalties were clearly "right." It felt easy to dismiss the cautions and concerns of people inside and outside of the work.

Still, there were chinks in the armor. The negative consequences of an exclusive emphasis on criminalization had been meticulously documented and compellingly argued for years. Beth E. Richie laid out the intersections of racism, prosecution of poor Black women, and domestic violence in her groundbreaking book, *Compelled to Crime: The Gender Entrapment of Battered Black Women* (Routledge, 1995). Tillie Black Bear, director of the White Buffalo Calf Woman's Society in South Dakota, and the women of Mending the Sacred Hoop in Minnesota demonstrated the connections between the forced removal of Native American children and the rise of family violence on reservations. For decades they argued for the restorative-justice tactics of health care, economic development, alcohol and drug treatment, and reparations instead of longer prison terms. Advocates working in lesbian and bisexual women's communities in Seattle collected evidence to demonstrate that, in one year, over half of the lesbian survivors who had come into contact with the police had been arrested. These advocates argued for more community-based solutions that did not rely on prosecution and incarceration. South Asian, Eastern European, and Pacific Islander immigrants articulated the connections among harsh and confusing immigration policies, the increase in the trafficking of women and children into the United States, and their experiences of abuse.

Attorneys called for greater assistance in civil legal issues, since domestic violence survivors are far more often caught up in civil matters like custody battles than they are in criminal cases. Still other activists showed how the movement's immersion in an adversarial legal system was dehumanizing people who batter and costing us opportunities for grassroots community involvement. As advocates spread the message that people who batter are fundamentally criminals, friends and families become increasingly hesitant about getting involved. As a result, it grew harder to undermine the isolation of abuse.

In these critiques, people were calling for greater complexity in our thinking and our work. In the domestic violence field, as in almost every movement to make justice and stop human suffering, the urgency of the need can narrow our view and disorder our priorities. We can convince ourselves that the harm we are trying to end is so bad that the details of how we stop it don't matter.

The movement to support women's self-determination and end family violence started down the path to criminalization with the intention of seeking justice and creating a societal stake in women's safety. By paying too little attention to the complexities of the issue, it found itself floundering in an ever-urgent, perpetual-crisis maelstrom of criminal legal response. The work required to build and sustain this response consumed most of the movement's resources, diverting energy away from community-based strategies that took into account the limits of a criminalized response. As a result, the movement inadequately addressed the concerns most expressed by survivors—breaking isolation, building community support, meeting children's needs, and fostering economic stability.

Minimizing

> I minimize with myself. If anything happens, I'm like, "Well, I didn't get shot, so what do I have to complain about?"
>
> Community organizer

I was working with the Audubon Nature Institute in New Orleans 10 months after Hurricane Katrina. Its programs include the zoo, the aquarium, and multiple learning centers and parks throughout New Orleans. A gentleman who had been dedicated to caring for the animals during and after the storm had eventually gone to visit his sister on the East Coast. He was walking with her on a city street when they encountered the body of a man who had fallen from high scaffolding and died just as the medics arrived. As they continued on, his sister admitted that she was extremely unnerved at his lack of reaction to what they'd just seen. "How could you not be shaken up or show any emotions?" she asked.

He told me, "On the one hand, I felt like I should explain to her, and on the other hand, I felt kind of defeated. I thought to myself, 'She can't understand, she won't get it.' I've seen so much in these past 10 months that I just don't feel much deeply anymore. I didn't know how to communicate that to her so she'd understand." He said he could not imagine what would have to happen for him to experience strong feelings again.

People who bear witness to a range of human experience may become increasingly inoculated to others' pain. We may start out being moved by each person's story, but over time it may take more and more intense or horrific expressions of suffering to deeply move us. We may consider less extreme experiences of trauma as less "real" and therefore less deserving of our time and support. "Minimizing" occurs when we trivialize a current situation by comparing it with another situation that we regard as more dire.

Minimizing is not triaging and it is not prioritizing. This coping strategy is at its worst when you've witnessed so much that you begin to downplay anything that doesn't fall into the most extreme category of hardship. While you may still be able to nod and do active listening and feign true empathy, internally you are thinking something like, "I cannot believe this conversation is taking 20 minutes of my time. There wasn't even a weapon involved." (Figure 4.11)

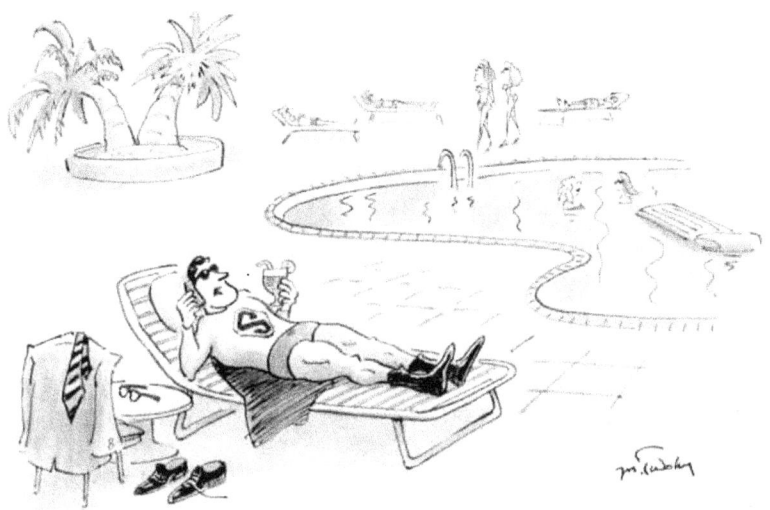

Figure 4.11: "Listen, pal, they're all emergencies."

It takes only one extreme situation to get us started on minimizing everything else. Again, minimizing is not setting priorities in our work, it is the experience of losing our compassion and ability to empathize because we are comparing others' suffering or putting it into a hierarchy. We may also begin to minimize when we feel saturated to the point that we can't possibly let any more information in. Instead of being able to experience the given situation for what it is, we minimize what we are hearing or seeing. We do so in a desperate attempt to avoid hitting our breaking point. We are literally at capacity.

This phenomenon is frequently a factor in creating a negative organizational culture. If only the most extreme cases deserve attention or get respect, then it behooves us to experience and express things in the most extreme way, right? Related to this, if we are voicing our irritations, concerns, and even legitimate critiques in very escalated ways, it is difficult for people to come to us with a complex response, and soon everyone may wind up taking sides. For example, if a worker says, "I feel like my boss just beat me up," it's much harder for anyone to talk through the specifics of the conflict than if the worker had said, "I do not feel that my objections were taken seriously, and I felt like I was being railroaded into agreeing to this task."

Finally, comparing leads to competition. If it takes something extreme to catch everyone's attention, well, we can meet that challenge! We may pump up the drama, or we may want to mine for the extreme in a situation so that our caseloads or issues seem more legitimate. Then we can have the prestige of being a person who handles the "real" stuff and who works for an agency that really "gets it."

Many people report that minimizing causes great distress in their personal lives. For example, your partner comes home from work and starts to describe his hard day, and you respond, with teeth clenched, "Really, honey? A hard day at your dot-com job? Sit down, and let me tell you about people who have hard days." Or your children pour out a story about something that upset them on the school playground, and you reply, "You should be grateful you get to go to school and have a playground at all. Do you know how few children around the world have playgrounds to play on?"

One family caseworker told me this story involving her five-year-old daughter. The child approached her mother for help with a mild, yet sincere, grievance about her father, only to be met with this explosive response: "You're lucky you even have a father. Every day I work with kids who don't have a father. Have never met their father. Don't even know what a father is!!!" Mortified at her sudden and impassioned outburst, the caseworker tried to undo the damage with her daughter but found in subsequent weeks that it had made an impression. Her daughter would repeatedly ask her, "Mommy, do you think that little boy has a daddy? What about that little girl?"

There may come a point when you feel as if nothing, ever again, will engage your empathy. A teacher once told me that she'd had days when her children would begin to complain about something and she'd retort, "It's not Auschwitz." That would be the end of the conversation.

Chronic Exhaustion/Physical Ailments

> I feel like I need a wheelbarrow for the bags underneath my eyes.
> AmeriCorps worker

I feel like I need a wheelbarrow for the bags underneath my eyes.
AmeriCorps worker There is a difference between feeling tired because you put in a hard day's work and feeling fatigued in every cell of your being. Most of us have experienced a long day's work and the reward of hard-earned exhaustion. We sink into bed grateful for our soft pillows and the promise of a sweet night's sleep. That is one kind of tired. The kind of tired that results from having a trauma exposure response is a bone-tired, soul-tired, heart-tired kind of exhaustion—your body is tired, your mind is tired, your spirit is tired, your people are tired. You can't remember a time when you weren't tired. (Figure 4.12)

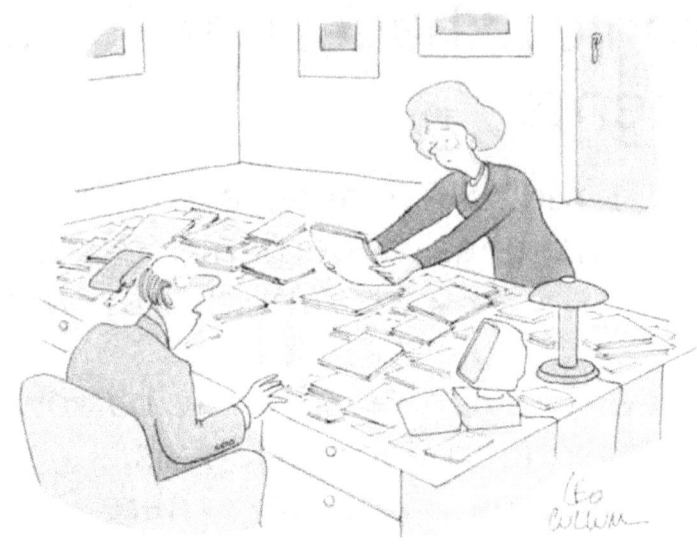

Figure 4.12: "No, not there, please. That's where I'm going to put my head."

This kind of exhaustion is most likely to emerge among people who feel completely overwhelmed by the urgency of the tasks at hand, but it also affects workers who have a balanced sense of what they can and cannot accomplish. Kati Loeffler is a veterinarian and scientist based in China. Her work includes improving the quality of care of domestic animals, working in wildlife conservation, doing veterinary and husbandry training in a giant panda breeding center, providing veterinary care for a black bear rescue center, and working to improve animal welfare and protect natural habitats internationally. "It is difficult to say how much of one's weariness and compromised energy and the struggle against despair are due to one's personality and aging body and how much to the toll of one's work," says Loeffler. "The extent to which animals suffer, as individuals and as species, due to human activity is overwhelming, and what little the handful of us who are trying to protect them from our own species are able to achieve is so very little and so very slow. Realization of the overwhelming need and pain in the world and our relative ineffectiveness to mitigate it is difficult to cope with."

Trauma exposure itself is tiring. As exposure accrues, our bodies and minds will require extra attention in order to become fully rested and refreshed. The situation becomes even more difficult if we get stuck in a trauma exposure response. Our symptoms, like feeling helpless and hopeless or being hypervigilant, are exhausting in their own right.

One underrecognized factor that may contribute to our level of fatigue is the belief that we have no choice about the work we do. This understanding may be conscious or unconscious. We may tell ourselves that we have no choice because our task is too important—the fate of the planet rests in our hands. Alternatively, we may feel bound to our work without knowing why. For example, it may never have occurred to us that our lives have been shaped by a deep-seated conviction that given our family, our ancestors, our destiny, there is no other work we can do. Even if we think we could change jobs, we may believe that we're meant to remain in a helping profession. When humans feel obligated, they very often feel tired.

Additionally, I know that in many fields, a sense of fatigue can become an accepted aspect of a seasoned worker's demeanor. Many of us are familiar with the "been there, done that" ethos that takes root in workers when they've been on the job or in a particular movement for a while. Compared to the cynical, world-weary old-timers, people who are excited and energetic are often seen as young and naïve.

The fresh-scrubbed and hopeful idealism of the new worker starting out may gradually give way to a thrashed, haggard, martyred persona. This persona conveys that you are too cool for immature optimism, that you have been around the block and have seen a few things, and that you are important—and this persona can actually be contagious. In the Pacific Northwest, for example, it's often gray out, there's coffee all around, and when everyone says "I'm tired" during the check-in at the beginning of staff meetings, it can be easy to just go along, knowing that if you express any high level of energy at all, you may be accused of being manic.

> I don't have energy for anything anymore. It literally takes all my energy to get up and try to just walk the dog, let alone do anything else. You don't even have energy anymore for the things you enjoy doing. Doing anything at all just feels like too much.
>
> Domestic violence worker

Finally, we can try so hard to keep from hitting rock bottom that we feel exhausted from the effort. We may be so invested in minimizing and ignoring the many consequences of trauma exposure and proving that we are still up for any challenge that we push ourselves harder and harder. Instead of taking the break we need, we may take on another project or commit to another campaign—hoping that it will give us a boost to overcome our sense of fatigue. It's helpful to be able to discern if we're tired because of the accrued toll of many earnest days (or weeks or months) of work or if we are tired because we feel obligated, have internalized a persona of exhaustion, or are fending off that "rock bottom." Listening to our bodies is a direct way to gain insight.

As the Trauma Center in Boston, Massachusetts, writes in its literature for law enforcement officers: "Physical complaints are very common; the body keeps the score." Back pain, migraine headaches, body aches, clinical depression, high blood pressure, and other ailments may be symptoms not only of physical distress but also of the accrued consequences of trauma exposure. As I continue my work with trauma exposure, I increasingly hear stories of people for whom the physical impact has been severe. Dozens of workers have told me about newly diagnosed health concerns, including stress-induced diabetes, chronic fatigue syndrome, and cancer. A common theme is that they are being urged to take a leave from work by their doctor and yet they're having a hard time doing it. Recently I worked with a chemical dependency counselor who had no history of heart disease in her family. She told this story: "I grew up in an alcoholic family where at age seven I was responsible for my younger siblings. So when I am asked to do something, I am committed to doing it. At my job, a colleague left, and I was assigned her workload—temporarily, they told me, but a new hire never came on. Several weeks into carrying two full-time caseloads, I had a heart attack at work. When I came back to work after recovering, my agency was restructuring. When they delegated our new caseloads, mine was the exact same number of cases as before. I went to my supervisors and said, 'I can't do this.' They apologized and took away half of it, leaving me with the caseload for a full-time plus a part-time position. I tried to do that. Six weeks later I had my second heart attack. And it was only then that I was able to be clear that I can only do my job, and my job alone. But it was really, really hard for me to admit that." (Figure 4.13)

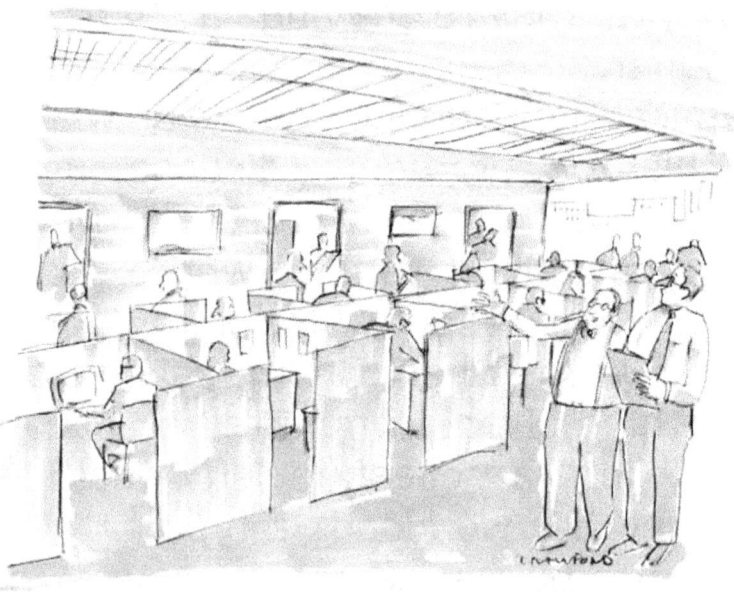

Figure 4.13: "And the dim fluorescent lighting is meant to emphasize the general absence of hope."

A DREAM REALIZED WARREN BROWN

WASHINGTON, D.C.

After graduating from Brown University in 1993, Warren Brown worked as a reproductive health educator in Providence, Rhode Island, and in Los Angeles. However, he soon became frustrated with the required curriculum, which did not answer the questions his students asked. He decided he wanted to combine a law degree with advanced public health training, so he went back to school. After his graduation from George Washington University in 1998, Brown took a job litigating health care fraud on behalf of the federal government for the Department of Health and Human Services.

Meanwhile, he pursued his personal passion for creating cakes. On New Year's Eve, 1999, he resolved to start selling what he baked. He maxed out his credit card to buy an oven, a double-door refrigerator, and other basic equipment. For the next 10 months, he maintained an exhausting schedule of full-time legal work followed by three to five hours a night in the kitchen. He quit his HHS job for good in 2000. Two years later he founded CakeLove, which features all-natural confections made from scratch, and which has repeatedly topped readers' polls as the best bakery in Washington, D.C. Brown has attracted a wealth of media coverage, even appearing on The Oprah Winfrey Show, *and in 2006 he was named the capital's Small Business Person of the Year. Brown continues to pursue his entrepreneurial spirit by opening additional stores, expanding the product line, and hosting* Sugar Rush *on the Food Network. He frequently speaks to young students and rising entrepreneurs about business development and finding one's passion. The following lessons for living were drawn from the testimonials he includes on his Web site,* www.cakelove.com.

Law school was a grueling period of endless projects and paperwork. I felt like I was losing connection with myself. Early on in the program, I was compelled to ask, "What makes me happy?" Asking myself this was key. It helped me take control and salvage my graduate school experience by setting aside time to do good things for my soul. Looking back, school wasn't the enemy; it trained me to focus. And even though it felt like a creative straightjacket at the time, I funneled loads of extra energy into very satisfying creative moments. Together, they got me to my passion.

Something forced me to face and examine the question, "If not now, then when will I make my move?" I felt like I was bobbing: not going under, but also not going anywhere. My mind and body wanted to express themselves, but, in adjusting to life in D.C., I just did not see a venue from which to perform. After a year of grad school, I realized I would have to create my own world of satisfaction.

In an effort to find satisfaction, I listened to myself. I asked myself questions and listened to my responses. At that time, my questions were all over the place, really scatterbrained. I tried to let everything that even hinted at being a response find its voice. Over time, this voice manifested itself in different ways: cooking, drawing/writing, gardening, yoga, etc. I tried as many new things as I could.

One of the most difficult hurdles I faced in understanding how to vent my soul came during a summer internship in law school. I abruptly left the internship after only four weeks of work. I've always had mixed feelings about leaving: I didn't want to fail to complete a job, but I wasn't happy and saw no hope. While figuring out whether to leave the position, I turned to drawing as therapy. One of my drawings was a self-portrait—a young man with an ashen gray face, blue lips, reddened eyes, and wilting hair. Bleak and miserable for sure. Drawing this image was clear and convincing evidence that something was terribly wrong. The next day, I left the internship.

Of course, friends and family were shocked that I quit, but many people congratulated me. How odd, I thought. I wasn't so sure why I should be congratulated for leaving a position, abruptly at that, and moving on to nothing except soulful self-indulgence. They saw me taking a step towards something that would make me happy. But I wasn't sure I could see what made me happy. I only saw what didn't make me happy. It turns out, of course, that half of knowing what you want is knowing what you don't want.

Perhaps part of that experience demonstrated to me that it is possible to leave something without an absolutely fixed idea of what the future will hold—as long as you are following a passion toward a productive end. It was a difficult lesson, but perhaps one of the best yet. I relied on this experience four years later, when I planned my exit from practicing law to develop my cake business.

Confident that my world would not collapse if I took matters into my own hands, I made some resolutions. I believe in making resolutions—practical ones that have merit help me. I allow myself all the time that I need to identify and understand what a resolution should be. I work to maintain and revise former resolutions so that I'm consistent and not constantly reinventing myself.

In 1999, I was struck with tremendous clarity in developing a set of resolutions: direct yourself to greatness; answer your calls; answer to yourself. This became my mantra, a meditating chant, a testament to end each day with, or juice to push myself further. This was the same year that I resolved to start baking. I wanted to expand my knowledge and skills in the kitchen. Measuring my triumphs and tragedies in the kitchen was easy. Coming to grips with the "big three" was a bit more of a challenge.

DIRECT YOURSELF TO GREATNESS. Sounds a bit haughty,

maybe? It's not meant to. It's about obeying priorities. I envision my idea of success, and just as if my body is a puppet, my mind is the puppeteer that commands my body to act and make the vision happen.

ANSWER YOUR CALLS. Literally taken from an effort to stop evading phone calls in a period of my life when I felt morose and antisocial, this precept is really a commitment to venting my soul. Lending an ear to my inner voice, my id, the kid in me, my instincts. It's a commitment to not abandoning the hope and expectation that I have value—and I'll see it when I direct myself to greatness.

ANSWER TO YOURSELF. To thy self be true. At some point during graduate school, I became passive. I began waiting for events to happen rather than making them happen. Eventually I realized that I could continue asking myself what I want out of life for the rest of my life but not experience the main event: feeling alive. Once I refused to ignore the fact that big chunks of my life would slip right by if I didn't seize control and move, I began to discover my passion. I took a leap and threw cake parties. This is how CakeLove started. I hosted cake open houses to launch and publicize my business in its very early days. I knew I had a knack for baking, I enjoyed hosting parties, and I wanted to survey a crowd for support of my venture. It was not easy to put myself out for review by the public, both for a critique of the quality of my baking and for an assessment of the viability of my plans. Many people told me I was crazy to leave law to bake cakes. And most did not understand what kind of cakes I planned to market. But my legal training helped me identify a ripe market niche as well as develop solid recipes. I felt like I was on a mission to bring together everything I had ever learned. It was very difficult, but I also loved it. (Figure 4.14)

Figure 4.14

Plain and simple, passion is a commitment without condition. It requires intensity for caring about something without regard to difficulty. It's a lot like love. Passion has meant finding myself happy baking cakes at 1:30a.m. at the end of an 18-hour day, or occasionally smiling while scrubbing cake pans because it means business is still growing. It is a choice to take a chance where the work is left to you. Everything about passion can be hard at times. But the benefits and rewards for indulging it simply cannot be measured. Both the good and the ugly experiences I've had have helped me grow, and for that I am thankful.

And that's what finding a passion is all about: you. Do you want to fast-forward to the answer? Try not to. The best parts of life are in the roads traveled to get to your destination. That's where you struggle and that's where you laugh. Be in the moment and enjoy it. Taste life. Taste what interests you. Listen to yourself and the world around you. It's a slow and tedious process where being patient helps a lot. Take your time to be sure of what you want. Then work like hell to get it.

Being passionate is about recognizing what makes you happy, focusing on and learning about it, and, ultimately, doing it in the name of your own satisfaction and pleasure. It's not self-centered to lead your life in a direction that satisfies you. It's necessary to feel at peace. Prioritizing your passion means that you carve out room in your life to explore and understand it. Once you understand yourself and what you care about, you'll be in closer touch with your life and the others around you. For a while others may see you as aloof, but once you arrive at being in touch with your heart and soul, others will find inspiration in you to do the same.

How did it work for me? I explored my interests, developed them, listened to feedback, and kept going. Now my career is my former side interest and I love my job. Once I gave priority to what makes me happy, my life very naturally evolved into CakeLove. In April of 2000, I pushed too hard in too short a time span. It was too much, and on a seemingly random Tuesday in the very early morning, I lost the energy to keep going. Alarmed, I called my parents and told them I couldn't move my limbs. They would work if I really concentrated, but I could hardly focus on breathing. Confused, tired, and desperate, I called my wonderful neighbor, Karen, and asked her to drive me to the emergency room. At discharge from the ER, the doctor said to me, "You're fine, but you're not 15 anymore. You're suffering from exhaustion. Slow down."

I didn't think exhaustion could happen to me. But it did, and I felt

> the effects of that episode for months. Fatigue would set in and tell me loud and clear to "stop, rest, and sleep." But don't worry, these days I'm much better about keeping a close eye on how I'm doing, and I have plenty of help at the shop! In living my passion, when I wake up, I'm all go. I'm spiritually amped—ready and willing to dive into the satisfaction I get every day from baking.

Inability to Listen/Deliberate Avoidance

> I leave my voice mail box full.
> Nurse

When avoidance is a regular habit in your life, the highlight of your workday is when you don't have to do your job. When you go on home visits, you knock softly, you fervently hope that the jeep won't be repaired so you can't visit the research station, and you pray for inclement weather so you can have that long-awaited snow day. While voice mail was a good tool for avoidance, text messaging and e-mail are even better, since they provide that much less human contact. (Figure 4.15)

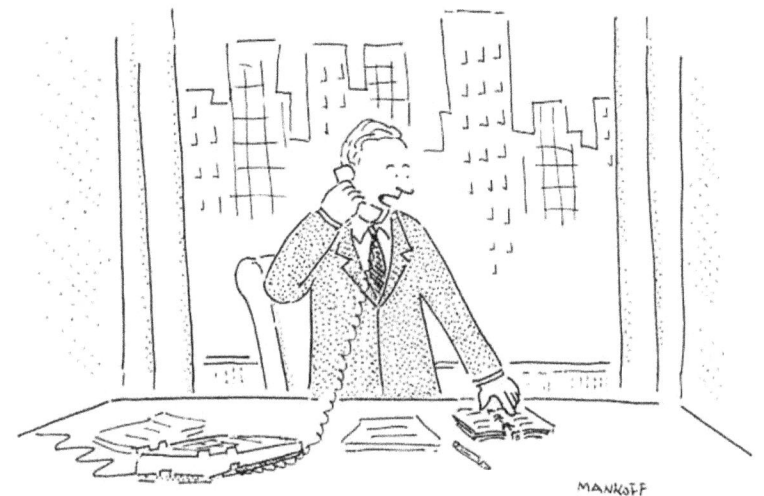

Figure 4.15: No, Thursday's out. How about never—is never good for you?

Now and then, when you get an unexpected break in your day, it makes sense to delight in the time and space that opened up—after all, perhaps you really are in one of those challenging positions where only if something cancels could you possibly get your stats done or your reports completed. And yet it is important to be aware of avoidance, because it can indicate that you are heading toward a much larger problem.

Avoidance often shows up in people's personal lives. You choose not to answer your phone. You go out with people less and less—and if you do, it's with a specific group of folks who "get it," or else it's with people whom you're confident will engage with you only superficially. Many people start feeling overwhelmed by their personal lives and lose energy for those things that once brought them joy: friends, family, yoga, sports, dancing, art, going out in general. As one attorney who did low-cost family law work recounted, "I never answer my phone at home anymore. My son got upset with me and said, 'Mom, what is your deal?' I said, 'No one I work with answers their phone at home.' 'That still makes you crazy,' he told me." This is one of the signs of avoidance: If we let others get close to us, it's often others who are avoidant at the same levels we are, so we feel justified in our behavior and don't see it as problematic in the least.

When I first started doing crisis intervention work, I used to be so excited to answer the crisis line when it would ring. Then it got to where I'd just watch the phone ring and I'd feel dread and I'd no longer pick it up on the first ring.

AmeriCorps program coordinator

Dissociative Moments

I can see the people trying to get across that bridge just like I can see you right in front of me. I close my eyes and I can see the people who died.

R. Omar Casimire, educator, artist, poet, and post-Katrina reconstruction volunteer

At Harborview Medical Center as an ER social worker, I worked with a family that had experienced such a tragedy that I could not speak about it at home for days. I could not get any distance from the story, the images, the smell, and the sounds. When I finally began talking about it with my partner, he listened attentively and took in the details. We had been driving and now we had stopped to go into a store. As

I continued the terrible story, I slowly realized that for the past few minutes he had been backing into a parking spot and then putting the car into first gear and moving forward. Backing in, putting the car in first, moving forward, again and again. I stopped my story and said, "Sweetie, what are you doing?" He looked at me, surprised. "Nothing, I'm just parking the car." This is someone who has heard his share of trauma and is extremely skilled at debriefing, but for some reason, in that instance, he became dissociated and wasn't even aware of parking and reparking the car.

A dissociative moment can happen when a person experiences intrusive or overwhelming feelings. It is the experience of being engaged in your work and, for whatever reason, having something suddenly unhinge within you. You realize that you have not heard the last five sentences of what someone just said, or maybe you failed to track the behavior in front of you; you're not following the story at all. Instead you're remembering the last injured animal you couldn't save or the day your brother became incarcerated or the time when your child was very ill. These are common occurrences. They are problematic only when we try to be stoic and plow through by pretending our reactions aren't happening.

We may externalize our feelings, imagining it's the client's fault that we feel so bad, or we may internalize a sense of worthlessness because we're having them. If we're so jacked up by what we're hearing, how can we possibly help others?

It is important to remember that any organism exposed to trauma will try to protect itself as a matter of course. In dissociative moments, we cut ourselves off from our internal experience in order to guard against sensations and emotions that could be overwhelming to our system. The *Newsweek* article discussed in the introduction contains an example of this phenomenon: "Like many others who work with the VA system, Bob Schwegel is a veteran himself. He helps Iraq vets apply for benefits, but it's tougher and tougher for him to continue as he listens to their stories. 'I get flashbacks of Vietnam. Sometimes I have to just get up and walk away.'"

Anyone with a personal history at all related to the work they do is likely to have experienced such dissociative moments. Many workers without a personal connection also report having such experiences, often for reasons they cannot explain. No matter who you are, these moments can be expected when you are exposed to others' suffering. It is important to notice them, avoid isolation, and seek out the support you need.

Sense of Persecution

> What if you can't do anything different? I'm in my fourth year of residency. What if leaving isn't an option?
>
> Family medicine resident

For our purposes, feeling persecuted speaks to feeling a profound lack of efficacy in one's life. We become convinced that others are responsible for our well-being and that we lack the personal agency to transform our circumstances. This notion has less to do with our physical surroundings than with our internal state. We may believe that we deserve better pay, safer work environments, more respect, adequate time away from work, and greater resources, and all this may be true. We can begin to seek change and reform in ways that are earnest, ethical, and fully committed. Alternatively, we can succumb to a belief that we have no capacity to influence any outcome. If so, we consent to suffer and relinquish power over our personal experience to outside forces. For many, this belief system may be inherited. As one social services director said, "Look, I come from a martyr heritage. Both my wife and I; I mean, martyrdom is what our families are all about."

Mistreatment can become a self-fulfilling prophecy. We may seek it out, focus on it, and then chalk it up as further evidence of how wronged we are. It can get to a point where our sole motive in identifying persecution is to locate more proof that we are being exploited. And of course, we do live in a world that is rife with oppression and mistreatment of living beings and our planet. We never have to look far for examples. When we talk about a sense of persecution, we are talking about a state in which individuals, and eventually organizations, begin to thrive on choosing to remain powerless in the face of adversity. James Mooney, a medicine man of the Seminole Nation, is fond of the saying, "The person who wins the battle is the one who doesn't show up." He isn't advocating that you should not show up for your life, but rather that you should be present in a way that refuses to engage antagonistic, reactive energy. There is often a clear path around our obstacles if we allow ourselves to back up, untangle ourselves from the brambles, and find another way. (Figure 4.16)

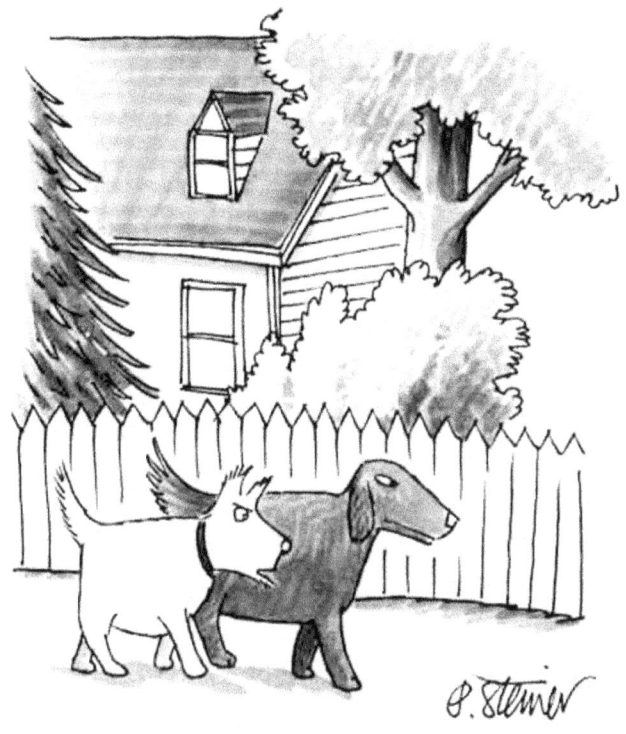

Figure 4.16: "It's always 'Sit,' 'Stay,' 'Heel'—never 'Think,' 'Innovate,' 'Be yourself.'"

This other way is illustrated by individuals and communities that have endured torment and brutality but remained in touch with their own inner strength. They have chosen to be powerful even in the face of persecution. A Holocaust survivor was asked to describe the horrors of being deprived of free will in the concentration camps. He said, "I had a great deal of freedom. I could decide if I looked up or down, if I looked to the right or to the left, if I put my right foot forward first or my left foot forward first."

It is not that having a sense of self-efficacy makes us immune to trauma exposure response, but it can give us many more options in terms of how we approach our life and make meaning of our experiences. Without a robust sense of being fundamentally in charge of oneself, a mindset of persecution can take root and we can lose faith in our own power to take the initiative. A community ecologist who worked in the Côte d'Ivoire after the civil war reflected, "The more common sequelae I see among my professional colleagues is an incredible inertia, something I would presume is akin to learned helplessness. So many loved ones, so many years, so many opportunities have vanished (for schooling, business, hopes for their children). Even with friends, in 'good times,' with resources flowing again, salaries, and normalcy, they seem unable to cope, to be proactive, to look forward."

I was struck by the discipline required to maintain a sense of personal agency during one of my graveyard shifts at Harborview Medical Center. It was three in the morning, and I was doing a psychiatric evaluation on someone who was in four-point restraints because he was having a psychotic break. He was calling me a bitch and trying to spit on me. The interview was taking longer than I felt it should. I wanted to get to my next patient, a sexual assault survivor. I began to feel persecuted and helpless, as if this man in restraints had all the control.

While I knew I had compelling reasons to feel overwhelmed, a disturbing feeling came over me: I was struck by how tenuous my sense of self-efficacy was. How quickly I could forget how deeply miserable anyone is who has to show up at the ER; how quickly I could lose sight of the fact that each person deserved my respect and empathy. It's important to remember that no one specifically needs to be doing the persecuting for us to feel persecuted. Out of the blue, forces may come to bear on us in a way that makes us feel powerless and done wrong.

When I meet with organizations, this often surfaces in the language the employees adopt to describe their circumstances. They may be public health workers using graphic war analogies to describe their feelings about reorganizations of their agencies or domestic violence advocates using battering analogies to describe their feelings about the treatment they receive from the board of directors. If we listen to our own comments, we can gain excellent insight into our state of mind with regard to self-efficacy and persecution.

Guilt

> I went shopping last week for a pair of shoes, and I thought to myself, "What kind of person would go shopping for a pair of shoes right now?"
>
> Community activist, New Orleans, nine months after Hurricane Katrina

Personal feelings of guilt are impossible to separate from larger forces like sociopolitical context, life experiences, and philosophical/spiritual beliefs. When we try to get a handle on guilt, we have to grapple with questions like these: How do we live in a world where there is such a disparity of resources? What can we do to neutralize imbalances? How do we participate in our own privileges in a responsible manner? And finally, how can I cope with this, enjoy my life, and not be immobilized by guilt? (Figure 4.17)

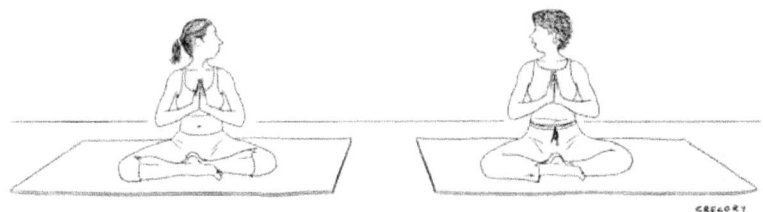

Figure 4.17: "I just found an Eastern philosophy that's very accepting of S.U.V.s."

There are a couple of things to note about guilt as it relates to trauma stewardship. One effect of guilt is that it can undermine the possibility for authentic connection between people. I was told by a chef who remained in

New Orleans after the storm that every time residents encountered each other, they would ask, "How'd you do? How'd you make out?" This was painful for him, he said. If they made out okay, he felt sorry for his own misfortunes rather than happy for them, and then he felt guilty for thinking that way. If the other person had lost more than he had, he'd feel sick with guilt about his relative good fortune. This comparison of suffering is counterproductive, because while it's an effort to connect in a loving and kind way, it often leaves the participants overwhelmed with guilt.

We can see a parallel process with a trauma exposure response when workers get caught up in their discomfort about the disparity between their lives and the lives of those they serve. In a distorted attempt to shield people from our privilege, or to minimize our privilege, we can begin to purposefully diminish our radiance and wellness, hoping to equalize the situation in the short term.

Diane Tatum, a longtime advocate for survivors of domestic violence, described returning on a Monday to the domestic violence shelter where she worked and being asked by one of the residents, "How was your weekend?" "It was fine," she answered, unenthusiastically. Which wasn't exactly how she felt, because she usually had great weekends and she had a great life, which, of course, was in part what allowed her to do the work she did. But she downplayed her happiness because she felt guilty that her life was going well, and she didn't want to flaunt it in front of people who were having a difficult time. Instead of giving an authentic answer, she hedged her bets and assuaged her guilt. In that moment, she distanced herself from the women at the shelter by not being genuine. Over time, we can internalize the flat "Fine" response and start to experience our life with less abundance and joy than we truly feel.

Back in the day in the domestic violence shelters where I worked, the survivors would remark that perhaps we, the advocates, should take time to do our nails or hair, as they did. It was a great statement that these women who had been through so much were still alive to the feelings of dignity and pleasure they could get from attending to themselves. Meanwhile, we as advocates were purposefully diminishing ourselves in an unsuccessful effort to connect with them more. Obviously we never want to flaunt the privilege in our lives: "Me and my husband who I'm legally married to and our big house? We had a great weekend!" It's just about being honest, not pretentious, not patronizing. It's about giving others the same honesty we'd expect if we were on the receiving end of services. It's about being real.

> I feel guilty because I can leave at the end of the day.
>
> Housing rights advocate

Guilt also interrupts our ability to take in and be present for the life-sustaining energy in our lives. Thich Nhat Hanh gives a talk in which he asks if we should have to work to appreciate the beauty in life. He replies that no, we should not ever have to work to take in what is beautiful, what is precious, what is sacred; we should simply be open to absorbing life's blessings as often as they present themselves. Because, as he says, "Suffering is not enough." Thich Nhat Hanh joins other masters who encourage us to be completely present for all things wonderful; if we are going to be present for life's suffering, we will need all the nourishment and rejuvenation that comes from life's beauty.

Guilt is one of the strongest signs of a trauma exposure response. It can block any experience of pleasure, peace, or happiness. Some workers find it difficult to enjoy a vacation (if they ever take one) because they feel guilty that they've left work behind while the habitats they're struggling to restore continue to be threatened. Others feel guilty about delighting in their children when they work with folks who, for whatever reason, aren't able to be with their children. Still others feel guilty living in a functioning community when they counsel clients who have lost their homelands to war. Workers have told me they won't explain that they're late to a meeting because their car broke down; they feel guilty for having a car.

Others will take off their wedding bands out of guilt for being in a relationship. Guilt is effective, then, in interrupting both our ability to be in the present moment and our ability to absorb all that is well in our lives.

One housing rights activist and shelter worker described the joy that can come from overcoming guilt and being authentic with our clients. He explained, "I like to cook, and one night I'd brought in some food I'd cooked. I felt guilty, though, so I was off in the corner eating and really trying to hide it. One of the residents came up to me and said, 'What do you got there?' 'It's nothing,' I said. 'No, really, that smells good. Did you cook that?' 'Yes,' I finally said. 'You know, I cook, too. I love to cook!' the resident said. Well, what happened then was I set up a way for us to cook together, and now we do that all the time. Not only that, but other men have come together, and there are cooking groups in the shelter. And you know, that's been really cool. That was never happening before."

Fear

> Fear is the cheapest room in the house.
> I'd like to see you in better living conditions.
>
> Hafiz, Persian mystic and poet

Fear can manifest in a number of ways: fear of intense feelings, of personal vulnerability, or of potential victimization. Fear is a natural and healthy response to much of what we witness. If we lived in a society where all people were supported in the full spectrum of their feelings, if there were no right or wrong feelings for a given situation, and if, when one felt fearful, one could simply share that with others, receive support, and move through it, fear would have a different impact. Instead, what often happens is that we live with a great deal of fear as a result of our exposure or hardship, yet we may not know how to process it, and thus it occupies space inside us. (Figure 4.18)

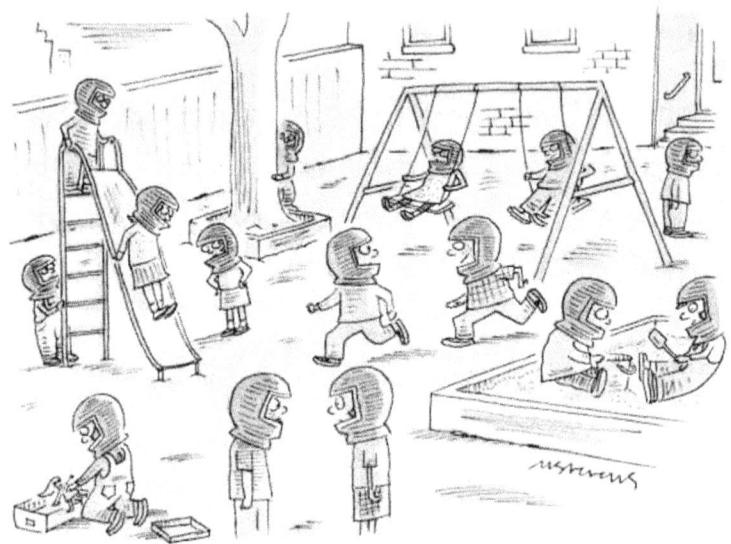

Figure 4.18: "I liked recess a lot better before the safety helmets."

Fear can squelch our ability to think creatively and well. As they said in the science-fiction film *Dune,* "Fear is the mind killer." Any number of damaging individual and societal trends have fear at their root. In the 1999 science-fantasy film *Star Wars: Episode I—The Phantom Menace,* Yoda describes the evolution of fear. He explains, "Fear is the path to the Dark Side. Fear leads to anger. Anger leads to hate. Hate leads to suffering."

Too many people want us to worry about too many things.

> I have a limited capacity for panic.
> It is not to be wasted on the trivial.
>
> John Petersen, Danish actor

Years ago, I was able to do some work with animal control workers, who were the most honest group I've heard from about this. With eloquence, they described how easily fear could harden into prejudices about certain breeds of animals, then morph into stereotypes about certain people, and finally leap into generalizations about races, socioeconomic groups, and neighborhoods. Whether the call involved neglected puppies or attacking dogs, they had to get on top of their fear. It is important to identify our fear and make the connections about what is fueling it.

One of the reasons it is hard for us to connect with our fear is that it makes us feel so vulnerable. It may make us uncomfortable to recognize that we have so much in common with our clients, who are also often fearful. If we are working to stop pandemics or racing against the clock to save the environment, we may worry that if we open the door to fear, it will completely overwhelm us, leaving us so swamped with terror that we can no longer act at all. In short, many of us opt to disconnect from our feelings of fear because it hits a nerve of our own fragility in life. Such denial may feel like the only viable path, but it is worth holding up to question. As we have noted, the physical price we pay for distancing ourselves from this natural response may be very costly.

When we acknowledge our own fear, we have an opportunity to deepen our compassion, not only for ourselves but also for every being that has ever been afraid. If we look deeply, many of us will discover that the fear that underlies all other fears is the fear of our own death. It is worth asking how we want to live knowing that we will die. The answer is generally not that we would quit. Rather, it is that we would embrace the preciousness of life. We would choose to be loving and compassionate, and to deepen our caring for others and the planet even in the face of our inevitable end.

Anger and Cynicism

When you see the suffering, when you experience it yourself, it's very hard to not want revenge.
Harn Yawnghwe, pro-democracy activist and director of the Euro-Burma Office, Burma (Figure 4.19)

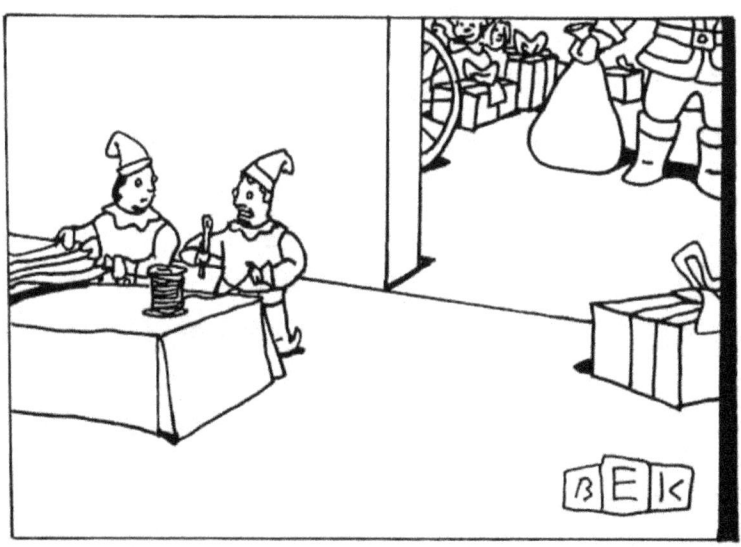

Figure 4.19: "Obviously, behind all the jolliness there's a lot of rage."

Anger is a common feeling among those trying to do right in the world. One may feel anger at the sources of injustice, at the treatment from one's organization, or at the clients themselves, to name a few. One may experience a hot, reactive anger or more of a cold, slow anger. Anger is complicated because the majority of people in our society have not been raised with good information or skills for managing it.

For most of us, anger is still primarily associated with times in childhood when bad things happened to us or when we had few concrete skills for channeling our feelings responsibly. How many of us feel like it's okay to feel angry? Do we know how our anger looks and feels to others? Do we know what's actually at the root of our anger? Do we know how to work with our anger and resolve it in a productive way that does no harm and instead results in creativity and positive change?

We can also look at anger from a framework of systematic oppression. From childhood on, there is often rigid socialization around anger: who is allowed to feel angry, who is expected to be angry, which groups are seen as angry people. These social norms most often fall along the lines of gender, race, and socioeconomic upbringing. For example, boys may be socialized to believe that feelings such as sorrow or fear may be more safely expressed as anger, while girls are often taught that it is socially acceptable to express just about any feeling except anger. In time, both boys and girls may lose their capacity to recognize or even experience the full array of their emotions.

> I have all this anger bottled up inside of me, and I feel like I can't let it out. I wouldn't know what to do with it, and I feel like it'd be too much. So it is just inside of me, and I can't hold it in anymore.
>
> Child protective services worker

We may be unaware of our anger, even when all of our loved ones, colleagues, and clients have to tiptoe around us. Years ago, I was asked to give a keynote speech on trauma stewardship to a large gathering of U.S. Air Force personnel. When we began talking about anger, I encouraged the participants to do a bit of homework once they left the conference. I asked them to connect with a loved one whom they trusted and say to that person,

"Tell me about my anger. Help me understand what it looks like, feels like, sounds like." I reminded them to not be defensive and to listen with an open heart and mind. There was widespread laughter. I said, "Hey, it's just a suggestion. Try it out." Several years later and thousands of miles away from that laughter-filled conference room, I was setting up to do a trauma stewardship workshop. A man who turned out to be in the Air Force approached me and said, "You know, I attended your talk several years ago and there was that section when you spoke about anger. When I got home, I asked my wife if she thought I was angry and what my anger looked like to her. It has completely changed our relationship. I actually think that I now have a sense of my anger."

If we are not comfortable with our own anger, our clients may find it impossible to process their anger with us. And there's another concern—we frequently take our anger out on people and animals and situations that are not connected to what our anger is actually about. They become our scapegoats.

Often when individuals try to deal with their anger honestly, directly, and in a good-faith way, it can be so unnerving for those around them that they may be viewed as "a bitch" or labeled intimidating. I am reminded of my father-in-law, who visits frequently. I often have the opportunity to hear him talking with his colleagues over the phone. Born and raised on the East Coast, he is able to communicate his various levels of anger effectively, without being passive-aggressive, pretentious, or needing to apologize for being straightforward. For me it can be unsettling; for him it's just Wednesday morning back East. (Figure 4.20)

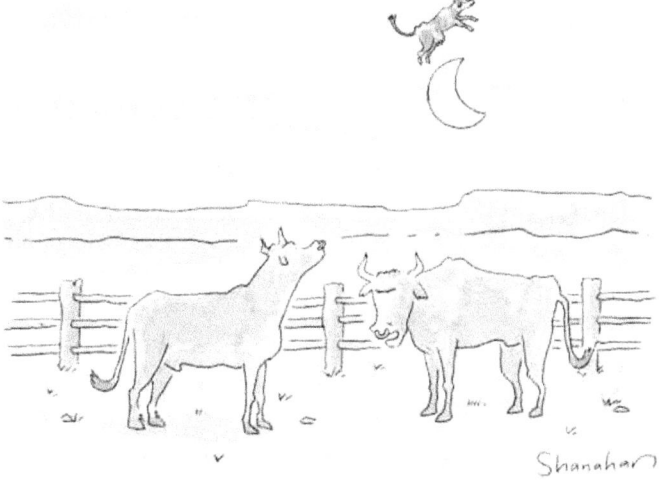

Figure 4.20: "But she'll come down eventually, and she'll come down hard."

I've heard many people say, "I'm not an angry person. We're not angry at our workplace. We don't have anger issues," and then they talk about how funny they are and how they're a cynical bunch. While anger is a natural feeling and in and of itself does no harm, cynicism is a sophisticated coping mechanism for dealing with anger and other intense feelings we may not know how to manage. Its undercurrent is anger, and yet it is often witty, quick, sharp, easy to laugh at, and incredibly alluring. Responsible humor is one thing, but cynical humor used to avoid dealing with feelings of anger is another. When cynicism is our main mode of humor, it can warp our sense of the world around us. As a character created by the American actress and comedian Lily Tomlin said, "I find it very hard to keep my cynicism up to the level of reality."

Inability to Empathize/Numbing

> I feel emotionally asleep.
> Executive director of an interpretation-services nonprofit

An inability to empathize with others, or feeling numb, often happens as a result of one's system being overwhelmed with incoming stimuli. Jon Conte, a professor of social work, clinician, and one of the forefathers of trauma exposure theory, says it is as if you are a sponge that is completely saturated and has never been wrung out. One can only take in so much. (Figure 4.21)

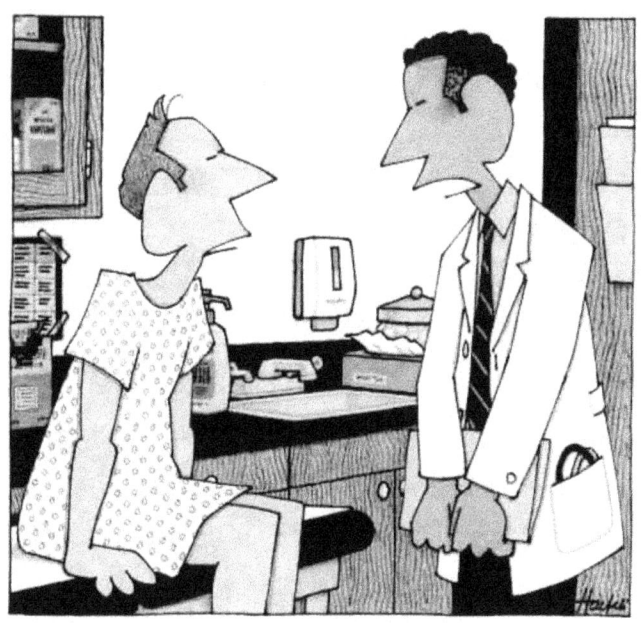

Figure 4.21: "Are you sure you're not confusing manic-depressive with awake-asleep?"

A pattern we often see is that people will get to a state of numbness, and their body and spirit and psyche will naturally try to regain a state of feeling. By now, we may have numbed out such intense feelings that any hint of experiencing them again, or of having any kind of a strong emotional response, may be scary or distasteful or leave us feeling out of control. We may find ourselves crying at a television commercial or yelling at our dog or having feelings that are real and yet not necessarily congruent with the situation at hand. One colleague said, "If I let myself feel this, I don't think I'll be able to pick myself up off the ground." And so we often welcome back the numbing and may even seek out ways to deepen it.

The body naturally employs a complicated mix of hormones and chemicals, sensory cues, and external stimuli to manufacture feelings. Feelings alert us to danger, aid in speedy decision making, focus our attention, and calm us down. We can override this system—that is, "numb out"—by amping up the production of feelings to the point that one is basically indistinguishable from another, or by shutting down the mechanisms for registering these feelings.

It goes from those "oh my God" moments when I used to read files to now they're just another file. You never wanted to get to that point where you lose that "oh my God" moment because these are really, really horrible things I'm reading.
HIV/AIDS caseworker

Numbing is not difficult. We live in a society and often work for agencies with innumerable mechanisms that encourage numbing. We have all experienced the urge to numb ourselves. As one conservationist and natural resources educator who works in Latin America and the Caribbean shared, "Conservation is a difficult field to be in. Your senses are flooded by knowledge and feelings of loss. You work with people who are constantly fighting and constantly feeling like they are losing. I myself am much moodier than I used to be. I have to drink sometimes, especially when I am away from home working. I'm not much of a drinker, but it helps numb my feelings when they make me anxious about how it isn't reconcilable."

Alcohol and over-the-counter, prescription, and street drugs are among the best-known tools for turning up the volume or shutting off the system. Similarly, overwork and overscheduling may cause our bodies to secrete adrenaline, a hormone that keeps us alert and racing around but may block our awareness of the feelings underneath. Dependence on caffeine and sugar may help us to feel better temporarily, but they also numb us to feelings of fatigue or craving.

> My children say I don't play with them anymore. I don't sing anymore, I don't laugh anymore.
>
> Family law attorney

In New Orleans I had lunch with Dina Benton. She is an extraordinary woman who lost her entire home in the hurricane and spent months driving around in her car, which was full of rescued possessions and her dog. She was one of the first civilians to return to her neighborhood after the storm, and several months later she got her job back with the Audubon Institute. She is now part of the team that will remain at the zoo, caring for the animals, should there be another severe storm.

When we met, Dina described the last 10 months of her life in a very even, rational way. As we were preparing to leave the restaurant, she ordered a cup of coffee and turned to me and said, with complete sincerity, "You know, that is one thing that I know is really different since Katrina. I drink around 14 cups of coffee a day now, and I never even drank coffee before. I have no idea why I drink so much coffee."

Whether from the rush of the amazing save or from a triple shot of espresso, once you know what it's like to be fueled by adrenaline on a consistent basis, it's hard to go back to a more measured and natural emotional state. We find that workplaces often adopt a very harried pace even when there's no crisis. Action for its own sake keeps people moving, makes them superficially productive, and limits their capacity for reflection about their lives.

This becomes seductive, even to workers, because we can confuse being amped up, attending to crises (some of which we create), and having a sense of being needed with being fully awake, living life, and being effective. It is interesting to hear what happens to people when they begin to slow down, pay attention to themselves, and take care of longer-term, root issues in their lives. Scott Douglas, an attorney and director of a volunteer legal services agency, shared this story with me recently:

> My partner and I both work for social service agencies; I run a volunteer legal program and he works with at-risk youth. We live in a huge old house with a great big yard, and we love puttering about, planting, pruning, and painting. However, there are always a million tasks to do on the house and yard, and anytime we're in any danger of running out, we make up new ones. Let's rip out this patch of lawn and reforest it with native conifers! That sort of thing.

A friend of ours lives across the street. One weekend morning he was leaning against his front door drinking coffee. He watched us scurry around like industrious squirrels hauling dirt and clippings, moving ladders, hanging laundry, mowing the lawn, planting flowers. Finally, he just shouted at the top of his lungs, "STOP DOING THINGS!" We were dumbfounded. What would that look like, not doing things? What would we do instead? What would happen to all the things we were not doing if we weren't doing them?

Workers have frequently told me about taking seven-day vacations and being sick for the first five days from an adrenaline crash. One person described having a panic attack "if I have more than two minutes alone in my apartment." A colleague once shared a story about how he and his wife, who had a managerial role at a hospital and who worked almost incessantly, took a vacation. For the duration of the week, she was unhappy. When he finally asked what was going on, she said, "You can't take me away for a week, strip me of all my coping mechanisms, and expect me to enjoy myself."

To allow ourselves to be carried away by a multitude of conflicting concerns, to surrender to too many demands, to commit oneself to too many projects, to want to help everyone in everything is to succumb to violence. The frenzy of our activism neutralizes our work for peace. It destroys our own inner capacity for peace. It destroys the fruitfulness of our own work because it kills the root of inner wisdom which makes work fruitful.
Thomas Merton, American Catholic theologian, poet, author, and social activist

Addictions

I look at my watch and see what time it is and how long until I can have a glass of wine. I mean, somewhere in the world it's got to be cocktail hour.
Human rights advocate

A colleague once told me that she had worked for an understaffed domestic violence program where the only acceptable reason for refusing to drop everything and come back in for a crisis was having had a few drinks. Alcohol, the organization reasoned, might impair the worker's discernment. "As a result, when the volunteers took over for the night, there was a sort of pell-mell rush as each staff member raced home to start drinking before our phones began to ring for help. Only drunk were you off the hook." (Figure 4.22)

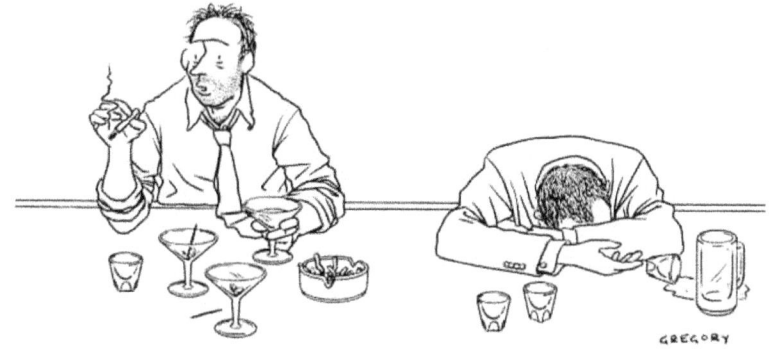

Figure 4.22: "Boy, I'm going to pay for this tomorrow at yoga class."

Of course, this is an extreme example. The point is that people can find themselves using drugs, alcohol, and other distractions to check out—both from a job's expectations and from internal messages. For some people, this tendency to numb out—whether by rushing home to drink or plugging into another violent video game or simply cultivating the ability to ignore your body's aches and pains—can graduate to addiction. There are many resources for help, and addressing the consequences of trauma exposure can help to lessen the fear of encountering the world in a feeling and present way.

An addiction is an attachment so strong that it persists despite our understanding of its potentially destructive nature. There are the classic addictions: drugs, alcohol, food, sex. But we can also be addicted to the rush of adrenaline—it's so tempting to stay wired when the alternative is to slow down enough to feel what is going on within and around us. There are so many ways to get hooked. It can be helpful to ask ourselves, "What am I most attached to? What do I count on to help me numb out? What would I be really resistant to giving up in my life?"

As the eighth-century Indian Buddhist scholar Shantideva once said, "We shrink from suffering, but we love its causes."

> I smoke two cigarettes whenever I leave the clinic. That's when I started smoking.
> Health care worker

An intriguing example of this is overwork, which for many of us becomes an addiction. It keeps our gaze down and our attention glued to our next step. We don't shift our gaze to observe the full range of what is in front of us. It can be hard and unpleasant to turn away from the sense of urgency we feel at work to focus on our personal life, where we may be held accountable as a peer, a community member, a partner, a parent, a son, or a daughter. Although people may not recognize it, the decision to work more and attend to their personal lives less is often a choice. One transitional housing worker shared, "My family is a real drain on me. I remind them that there are other people they can call on and other places they can go for support. I have enough to take care of with my work."

Our ego is a related addiction we often overlook, at least when it is linked to our culture of productivity-based identity. Many new stay-at-home mothers and fathers feel this when the rush of their work and its ego-boosting elements drop away. They're at home doing a job that is incredibly important to the world, and yet they feel as if they're not doing anything important at all. This experience is reinforced by a mainstream view that says, "We are what we do" and get paid for, not "We are simply who we are." (Figure 4.23)

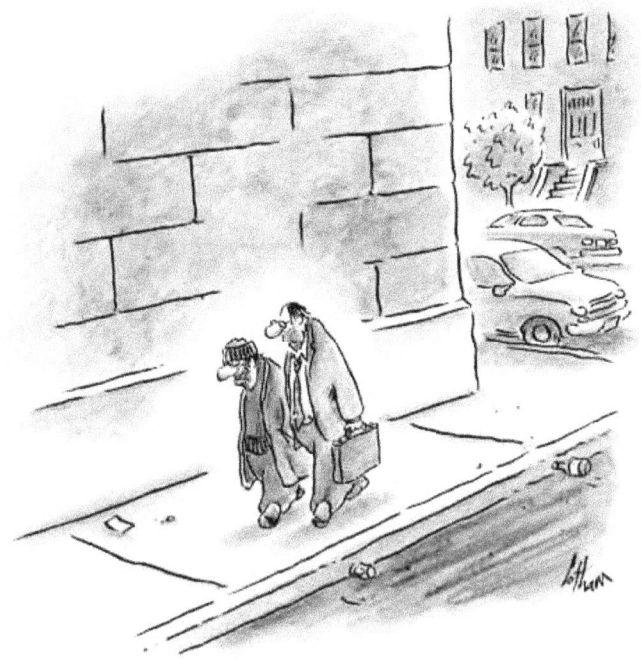

Figure 4.23: "I'm slowly weaning myself off employment"

Addictions can be particularly compelling for those whose work feels absolutely too intense to integrate. I once heard the word *equanimity* defined as "having space within for everything." Our internal space must be expansive enough that we can sit with the sorrow in life even as we can feel the miracle of it all. When our work is overwhelming, we can feel so overloaded that we don't have room for the pain and suffering of those we serve. What we have witnessed can feel like it is breathing down our necks, desperate to find shelter inside of us. As individuals and as a culture, we can become addicted to escape. When we believe that we lack the inner capacity to deal with our reality, we may seek out objects, activities, or relationships that will help us to perpetuate an illusion about ourselves, numb us out, or otherwise give us distance from overwhelming feelings.

While perhaps the things we use to block our experience are effective in the short term, over time we require more and more of them to effectively numb us out. At some point, the barrier we've tried to create against feeling our emotions is no longer adequately fortified by our addictions, and it ruptures. In comes everything we've been trying to avoid—but we're less equipped to deal with it than we would have been originally, because we invested in addictions instead of in sustainable coping skills.

Grandiosity: An Inflated Sense of Importance Related to One's Work

> Throughout the hospital, the only social workers who connected so strongly with their work, as if it was their total identity, were the ER social workers. They are the only group that if you asked them, every one of them would say, "I'm an ER social worker." It was their whole identity.
>
> Hospital administrator

When work becomes the center of our identity, it may be because it feeds our sense of grandiosity. This can be particularly challenging to acknowledge. Many people get hooked on involvement in others' lives: solving their problems, becoming a powerful figure for them, getting increasingly attached to the feeling of being needed and useful. The same dynamic may apply to people who are working with animals or the environment. If our work is breathtakingly important, so are we.

I have found that this form of grandiosity often keeps people in their work much longer than is perhaps best for them. You think, "Who else will do it if I'm not here?" or "I can't possibly leave, they're relying on me." While there may be some truth to this, it gets problematic when we're not firmly grounded in a larger reality. We need to acknowledge the value of what we bring without making our work be all about us. Once we cross that line, it can be difficult to come back. We can lose an accurate sense of our individual capacities and limits as well as our actual interdependence with others working in our fields. One animal activist said, "I am endlessly impressed by the stamina of some of my fellow animal rescuers. Although in some I recognize the telltale signs of the familiar rescuer messiah complex—the distracted movements, the permanent worry lines." (Figure 4.24)

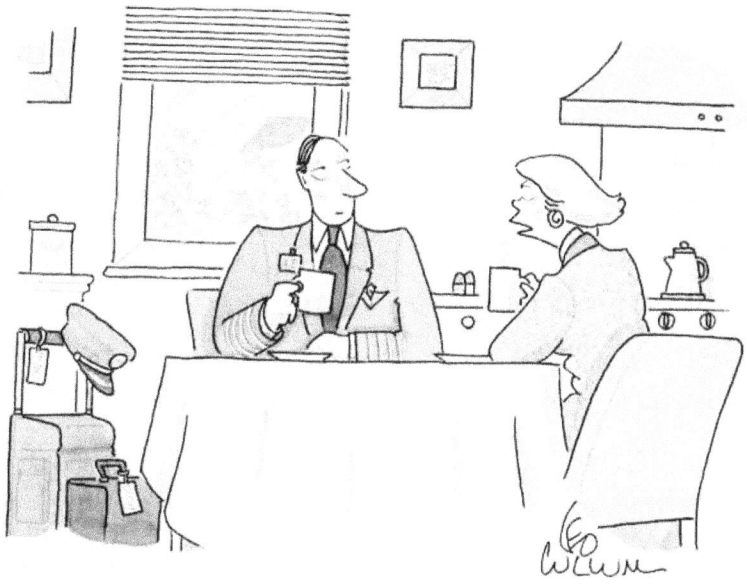

Figure 4.24: "Must you precede everything you say with 'This is your captain speaking'"

Admittedly, many people feel content with an identity based solely on work, particularly when that work is exclusively focused on others. Work gives us an excuse not to focus on ourselves, our relationships, or our lives, which may be precarious or falling apart. It is important to remember, however, that if we concentrate all of our energy on one area of our lives, we are likely to be compromising ourselves elsewhere. Ginny NiCarthy, a foremother of the domestic violence movement in the United States and the author of several revolutionary books on violence against women, described the tension she encountered when balancing multiple identities: "There I was, neglecting my own children while I was out trying to change the world."

Karyn Schwartz, an herbalist and a healer based in Seattle, Washington, describes why she sings. Despite the many demands on her time, she makes sure to perform as often as she can—in nightclubs, cabarets, and classical choirs. "A lot—maybe most—of what I do as an assistant to people's healing is invisible. I don't own anyone's well-being. If I am doing my job well, nobody feels that I am doing much at all, and I become quickly obsolete, because it's their journey, not mine. I sing because that is how I pray; I perform because I need to be applauded. All of us need appreciation, and sometimes in this kind of work the invisibility can start to feel depleting. In order to stay honest about my own need for accolades, and in order to nourish my own capacity to remain generous with my energy, I make sure to tend to the part of myself that needs to be a big diva. If I don't, I run the risk, as we all do, of relying too much on my work for my sense of esteem. When that happens, I can start to feel dependent on other people's suffering and their need for me to relieve it, for my own feeling of purpose. It's hard, in that dynamic, to honestly encourage someone else to be truly whole."

It can be very hard to reduce our identification with work, let alone break the addiction to overwork that often results. These ways of being are feverishly supported in certain societies. When I lived in Guatemala, I'd often be invited to sit with someone's family in a small indigenous community, high up in the mountains, and talk with them for hours. They posed many questions, but never once was I asked, "What do you do?" In Central America, Japan, Mexico, New Zealand, and throughout Europe, people ask where you live, how your family is, what crops grow near your home, what you think of their country, and so on, but not about what you do for a living.

Having been raised in the United States, where this is generally one of the top three questions we ask upon meeting new people, I marveled at what it means *not* to ask this question. In the United States, we are obsessed with work; it is a cornerstone of our self-image. This difference in perspective may help to explain why workers elsewhere in the world rarely exude the same exhaustion that we do in the United States. Perhaps their cultures make it easier for them to maintain a larger identity that is distinct from their work. Their understanding that what they do is not who they are may allow them a freedom that our grandiosity about work does not afford us.

PART THREE

CREATING CHANGE FROM THE INSIDE OUT

CHAPTER FIVE

New Ways to Navigate

> Chance has never yet satisfied the hope of a suffering people. Action, self-reliance, the vision of self and the future have been the only means by which the oppressed have seen and realized the light of their own freedom.
>
> Marcus Garvey, National Hero of Jamaica and founder of the Universal Negro Improvement Association and African Communities League

So far, we have traced trauma stewardship from our personal histories through the organizations where we work to the society in which we exist. We've peered into ourselves, identifying the effects of the accumulated, internalized stress from our work.

Now let us explore what we can do with our trauma exposure response. How do we alter our course to reach a healing path? How do we prevent the ripples of trauma exposure response from continuing to spread? How do we integrate the effects of trauma exposure so that we become effective trauma stewards?

For most of us, the answers to these questions won't come quickly or easily. More likely, you will face difficult decisions. The wonderful news, however, is that you already possess all the tools you need for this journey. More than anything else, what we need in order to practice trauma stewardship is knowledge of our own lives—what we feel, value, and experience, and what we need to do to take care of ourselves. The more deeply we can connect with ourselves, the more likely we are to find what we need to do our work joyfully and well, even in the face of significant hardship and obstacles.

The essence of the trauma stewardship approach is to cultivate the quality of being present, both to the events of our lives and for others and our planet. This most important step on the path to trauma stewardship is the same one that is said, in some traditions, to lead to full enlightenment. It is important to note, however, that you need not have a spiritual revelation to practice trauma stewardship. As the Tibetan Buddhist nun Pema Chödrön defines enlightenment, it is "whole-hearted, open-minded interaction with our world."

We all have the potential for this kind of interaction. Each of us can teach ourselves to be open, flexible, curious, and awake to our experiences. And once we accept this idea, no matter how paradoxically painful and challenging it may be to bring it to fruition in our life and work, it's like discovering that compass in our pocket that we forgot we had. As Peter Levine writes, "No matter how highly evolved humans become in terms of our abilities to reason, feel, plan, build, synthesize, analyze, experience, and create, there is no substitute for the subtle, instinctual healing forces we share with our primitive past."

While our deepest instincts are ultimately to do what is best for ourselves, sometimes we need guidance to recognize when we've wandered away from our truest selves, and lessons to learn how to regain our bearings.

As we map our trauma exposure response, we can shift into a more active phase of our journey—one that, as Marcus Garvey said, emphasizes action, self-reliance, and a new vision for our self and our future. In the remainder of this chapter, I will offer some general tips for the path you are about to travel. Although the questions and emphasis at each stage will be different, the basic approach remains the same. Remind yourself that it takes courage to undertake this journey, and practice compassion at every step.

Open the Inquiry

As we shall see, understanding where you are now may require that you look far back into your past. What events and decisions are most crucial to who you are today? Do you find any consistent themes as you look back over your choices? When I delved into my own history, I saw that my entire life had been shaped by a struggle to reconcile pain and joy. As a child, I was deeply preoccupied with the well-being of others and persistently troubled by the injustices in the world. When I was 10, my mother was diagnosed with a rare form of lung cancer, and when I was 13, she died. My brother and I were catapulted into adulthood. Although I was surrounded by love and kindness, I felt an isolation that was immense.

Throughout my childhood and adolescence, I searched for someone who could articulate my experience that there was a tremendous amount of suffering in the world even while there was a tremendous amount of beauty. I grew up far from the teachings of Buddhism; I was surrounded by well-meaning people who tried to soothe me by telling me that everything would be okay. Their comments left me feeling disconnected from what I instinctively perceived to be the essence of life: the complex coexistence of hardship and blessings.

When I was 18 and my professor of sociology was talking about homelessness, I experienced one of those moments when time stands still. As he told us that it was our responsibility to honor each other as humans to the best of our abilities, I felt a chord sounding deep within me. I went up to him after class and asked how I could start volunteering. I began my social work career in my freshman year of college as an overnight assistant in a homeless shelter. Being in the company of individuals who were suffering greatly and yet could tell a joke and laugh deep and hard resonated in me in a way that began to melt my isolation. My work expanded to child abuse, domestic violence, sexual assault, and trauma as a whole.

In graduate school, when it came time for a practicum, I felt moved by some larger force as I asked to be placed in a hospital trauma center—a place that was certain to bring up all my fears about grief and loss. Not long into my time at Harborview Medical Center, I realized that part of my reason for being there was self-serving. I was sharing in the human capacity to experience horror and beauty at the same time—on a daily basis, and on a massive scale. Even at the most devastated moments of their lives, people somehow called up their highest selves. They were suffering on a level I could relate to, and yet despite their anguish, they didn't give up. I received an infusion of awe and hope with each and every shift.

Over several years of graveyard shifts in this hospital, I felt my old isolation melt. Because I had the opportunity to bear witness to others' pain while helping them to know that they could be loved and taken care of as they suffered, I experienced a profound healing. My work at Harborview gave me a gift: a deep understanding of how I could struggle in my life and yet still be able to marvel at Mount Rainier and the Cascade Mountains during my run after each hospital shift. My patients taught me how expansive life is.

Years later, when I had the privilege of being introduced to Thich Nhat Hanh and Buddhism, I felt it all come full circle. This ancient tradition was deeply concerned with the relationship between suffering and joy that I'd grappled with since childhood and learned so much more about from my patients and clients over the years. Jack Kornfield, a Buddhist monk and educator, described Buddhism's central tenet when he said, "It's not easy. This human realm in which we have taken birth is halfway between heaven and earth, and it is said to have fundamentally an equal measure of suffering and pleasure, of joy and pain, of loss and gain, of the mundane and the daily punctuated by unspeakable beauty and oceans of tears."

You can understand how my work in the trauma center met my needs on some level. Before each shift I'd ask myself, "Given my understanding of the meaning this work holds for me, can I continue to be here, serve the patients well, and do right by them?" Each time, I decided I could, and I did, to the best of my ability.

My decision to leave the hospital came when it became apparent (well, my loved ones would tell you long *after* it had become apparent) that I could no longer stay on top of the enormity of what I was witnessing and experiencing and still serve patients well. At the end of my time in the ER, the accumulation of trauma had taken its toll. I did not yet have a daily practice of mindfulness, and I was no longer able to be present for what I saw and heard each day without losing faith in the larger workings of the universe. Even so, I was deeply connected to my work, and the thought of leaving tormented me. I confided to my mentor Billie Lawson, "No matter where I go, I'm never going to forget what I've experienced here or what it tells me about the brutality of life. So what does it matter if I leave or stay?" We were on a walk. She allowed a long moment to pass and then said firmly, "Laura, maybe you just don't need any more exposure." And so, when I was able to admit that I could no longer hold out the light and hope that the patients deserved, let alone personally maintain and engage in my own life, I decided it was time to leave Harborview.

I encourage you to ask yourself if what you are doing in your life is working for you on all levels of your being. Does it edify you? Do you use it to escape your life? Does it bring you joy? Does it support your ego? Is it a place where you can do something about the pain in the world? Does it distract you? (Figure 5.1)

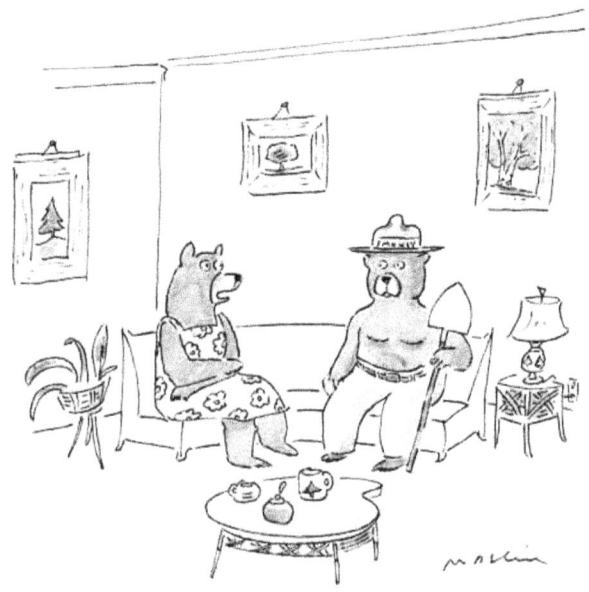

Figure 5.1: "Only I can prevent forest fires? Don't you think you should share some of the responsibility?"

I use my own story here as a tool to illustrate the strong, sometimes subconscious relationship between our self and our work, and how deep we may have to reach for the awareness necessary to bring the best of ourselves to the choices we always have. When I hit rock bottom and slowed down, I let go of my resistance to the possibility of change. As soon as there was an opening, fresh information and support, along with ideas for new ways of being, swiftly flowed in.

Practice Self-Care

Even if the answers to questions about your life's direction don't come instantly, there are certain practical steps you can take right away. You can begin by acknowledging that your stresses are genuine and you are looking for healthier ways to deal with them. As one disease ecologist who worked in Guinea shared, "For a long while, I didn't do anything to care for myself, as it took me some time to recognize that this was something treatable and 'real.' All I did was grieve for lost friends and listen to survivors' stories." By easing the burdens of trauma exposure, you may open the physical, mental, and emotional space to explore the deeper questions.

In his book *Psychological Trauma*, Bessel A. van der Kolk identifies important differences between those who are permanently debilitated by primary trauma and those who are able to integrate the experience into their lives and adapt. He finds several shared traits among "stress-resistant persons." Among them:

A SENSE OF PERSONAL CONTROL. Stress-resistant people perceive a connection between their own actions and how they feel; they believe in their own capacity to influence the course of their lives.

PURSUIT OF PERSONALLY MEANINGFUL TASKS. They are present and engaged in their lives, and this helps them to be active, instead of passive, during challenging times.

HEALTHY LIFESTYLE CHOICES. They show "decreased use or general avoidance of known dietary stimulants of refined white sugar, caffeine and nicotine; they seek out multiple periods of hard exercise each week; and, they find time each day for a period of relaxation."

SOCIAL SUPPORT. They have relationships with others who can serve "as a buffer in dealing with difficult situations."

Bessel van der Kolk concludes that stress-resistant people are "capable of negative affect when faced with adversity, [but] a belief in their actions to resolve problems results in a general mood of well-being." Just as there are noteworthy similarities between post-traumatic stress disorder (PTSD) and trauma exposure response, so too there is significant overlap between the coping strategies that best serve primary trauma survivors and the behaviors that can most benefit those of us impacted by trauma exposure through our work.

As we work with the Five Directions, we begin a practice that will enable us to bolster our resources in each of the four key areas of stress resistance that van der Kolk has identified. When we focus on north (creating space for inquiry) and east (choosing our focus), we enhance the link between thought and action and our sense of personal agency; when we turn to south (building compassion and community) and west (finding balance), we look for ways to create a culture of support around us and to make healthy choices that will serve to nourish our strength rather than deplete it. (Figure 5.2)

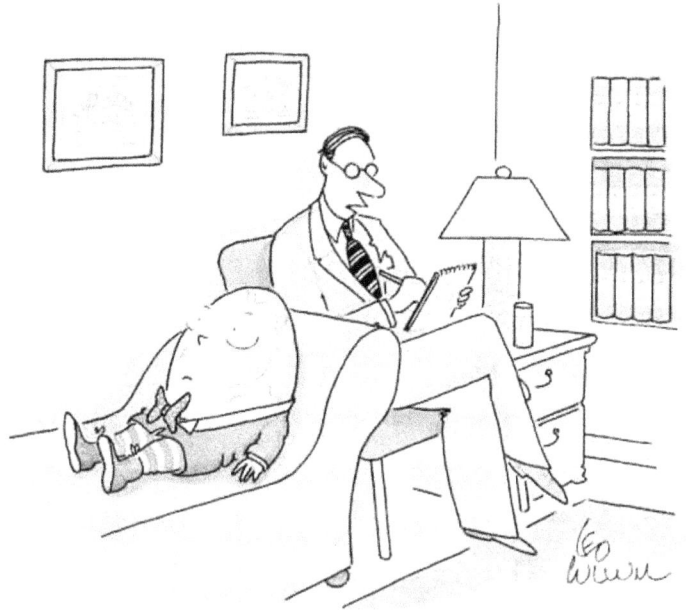

Figure 5.2: "Eventually, I'd like to see you able to put yourself back together."

It can be humbling to realize how much we have in common with those we attempt to help. Our pain and strategies for healing may look much the same as theirs. As caregivers, we too may find it nearly insurmountable to attend to our own well-being at times. And yet we face a challenge: How do we care well enough for ourselves to reconcile all that we are witnessing? Remembering how much we share with our clients, we might think about our clients' heroism, courage, strength, and determination. We can listen to what comes out of our mouths as we encourage, guide, or mandate them—and stop to wonder if we would be wise to follow the same advice. If we work with animals or plants or habitats, we may remind ourselves of all the ways that natural systems have evolved to keep themselves healthy and replenish themselves. If we think of birds, we may think of their urges to sing, to mate, to eat, to fly, to raise their young, to follow the rhythms of the seasons. If we honor this life in them, we can also attempt to honor it in ourselves.

Be Patient

I have heard countless colleagues express their despair, frustration, and disbelief that there's not a simple process to follow, a neat package to open, a timed-release pill, that will make all this better. These feelings of urgency and attraction to something quick and easy are, in and of themselves, a part of trauma exposure response. In truth, we *know* that transformation is a process. We *know* that the people, animals, and environments we're working with have a long road ahead of them. We *know* that our physical health requires daily maintenance, that we should do more than simply seek treatment once things go wrong. And yet when it comes to caring for ourselves while caring for others and our planet, we often choose to believe that, somehow, we are different. Somehow our capabilities must be greater. Somehow we are entitled to a less arduous, less introspective, less involved role in our own well-being. In fact, we are not. Trauma stewardship is based on age-old wisdom. It isn't necessarily fast acting—but it is reliable, trustworthy, accessible, and doable. It requires some trust that taking the first, and then the second, and then the third step matters. American civil rights leader Martin Luther King Jr. reminded us, "Take the first step in faith. You don't have to see the whole staircase. Just take the first step."

PROFILE DEADRIA BOYLAND

SEATTLE, WASHINGTON

CURRENTLY: Manager, the Community Advocacy Program, New Beginnings.

FORMERLY: Shelter program manager at a domestic violence agency for 10 years.

I was taught by my mother and father that you really have to take care of yourself, and also that taking care of yourself means being responsible. What that could look like is working hard, showing up every day, building that trust, so when you do need to take time off, people realize that you're not taking time off to just not come to work, but that you're taking time off to take care of yourself. And it's important that you work hard, have good structure and a good balance, so that when you're being affected by your work, you can see the signs and you can do things to take care of yourself.

When I'm affected by a woman's story or someone tells me something about a domestic violence situation, I can't stop thinking about it. I feel for that person. I think about them all day every day, and I can feel their pain. I know it's not the pain they feel, but in some sense I feel pain for them. I'm frustrated and irritated, and I want to fix it. I find myself calling back to work once I get home to see how she's doing or what's going on with the kids. I find myself moving into the advocacy role and away from the supervisor role; I start to switch roles and I realize it. I can see that transition happening, and I know that's not healthy, but somehow I manage to do it all. What I hear from other people is "Thank God you were here" or "Oh my God, I didn't think of that," which in some way makes you feel like you are doing a great job—but what it really means is that I've taken on someone else's trauma, and not only am I doing my job but someone else's job, too, and I start to realize that this is not healthy.

I can be a little compulsive in my work life and in my personal life as well. So being organized helps me realize when something is about to go down. I've realized that some staff are not so organized and may not realize how they're being impacted until they are sick, depressed, or really in the middle of a breakdown.

I don't know if people understand this, but when you're on autopilot and you're multitasking and you're not listening to what your body needs, like rest, a healthy meal, or laughter, this can be a result of trauma, and the way you deal with it can look different. You might show signs of depression, anger, avoidance, procrastination, or taking on too many things at once.

Being healthy and having a healthy lifestyle outside of work and having activities, that's what keeps me grounded. I could say that years ago it probably affected me more because I would stay at the shelter for 10 or 12 hours a day and come in on the weekends—it was my life. When I had a family, all that changed, and I put things in perspective. I realized there are things I can do and things I can't do, and I really think my solidness, my ability to be grounded, is what keeps everything else grounded. I can focus because I'm not bogged down by the trauma and the stress.

I think taking trainings on secondary trauma has helped [our agency] become well informed. Having someone from the outside who could work with us on trauma exposure has given us a clear perspective. Having monthly meetings where we can talk about situations that occurred on our shifts can provide support. This allows us to leave work at work and not necessarily take it home. Joining committees and networking with people who do the same kind of work in different agencies can help; connecting to people who I could talk to outside my agency but who could understand the work also helped. And I think the most important thing is recognizing that trauma exists, because if you deny that it's there, then you're suppressing it and not dealing with it. Being able to recognize it is huge.

There are a couple of things that I recognize as a manager. I recognize when we have a high-needs environment. I pay attention to the stories that women share, and I'm aware of how those stories will affect the advocates. I know there are some advocates who are going to be affected more because of their own histories with domestic violence, and I can see that coming down the pike. So I meet with them, talk with them, and touch base with them. I ask them how they're doing and feeling and ask if they want to talk, or if they need to take a walk.

Before each advocate starts her shift, she must debrief or overlap with the outgoing advocate. I'm adamant about the outgoing advocate purging before they leave. I want to be sure when they leave for the day that they don't take home the stress and trauma from the shift. And if that doesn't work, they can meet with me one-on-one. You can also do both, and that's always ongoing. That's always the process. They technically have 30 minutes, but I give them an hour to debrief if they need it, because they're still attending to the women and children in the program. I always tell them, when you leave here, you need to physically shake it off and walk out the front door.

I have very driven advocates. They work like there's no tomorrow. They are committed and dedicated. They believe in the work. Sometimes they are traumatized by the situations and the stories that they hear, but they continue to work together. I believe the reason why they work so well together is that I continually say to them, "We are a team." I tell them that if we don't work together as a team, we can't function properly. When an advocate leaves the program, I think about who will be the next team member to join us and how we can continue to keep this group cohesive. I believe that you have to work together, so you have to get along, like each other, and you have to support each other 100 percent. If I'm supporting you 100 percent, you have to give 100 percent.

In their personal insurance, our advocates have counseling resources. If you need to have time off, then request it and take the time. I respect them for taking their time off. I pay attention to their leave balance, because if I see that you're someone who is always using up all your leave, then I sit with you and ask what's going on. I want them to have the hours if they need them, but not deplete them.

I make myself accessible to the advocates. But they also know I'm going to hold them accountable. You can't just come to me and say, "I'm falling apart and I'm going to keep falling apart." They know I'm going to say, "Let's make a plan, and I expect you to stick to it, and I'm going to hold you to that plan," and I also support them every step of the way. I'm going to say to them, "This is what I notice; let me know what's going on so I can help you. It's not going to get better unless you talk about it. I can't fix it, only you can fix it, but I can support you." Once we have that conversation, the doors just open, and then I can help them navigate a plan that works.

I can sense when things are wrong, and I ask them to come into my office. I purposely sit in another chair, because I don't want them to see me as a supervisor but as a support person. Once they share what's going on, we create a plan and then discuss some options, and I ask what they'd like to do. Then I say, "We talked about it today and we're going to meet next week, and we're going to see what you've done." I hear from folks that they feel better, and then I say, "Oh, but we're not done. What's our plan for next week?" And we keep going until I feel like they have a better understanding about what's going on with them. I'm not doing the legwork, but I help them with their plan.

My thought is if they don't have a plan on how to deal with their trauma, then they can't do their work.

If they can't process what is happening to them personally, then it sits with them and pesters them all day long and they can't focus on being an advocate. By creating a self-care plan, they can begin to focus on their work, which is much like the women we serve, right? We must help the clients create safety plans and goals. We as advocates are helping others, but it doesn't mean we don't need help, too.

I have to be a leader. I have to practice what I preach. I can't say these things to them and ask them to follow a plan and hold them accountable if I'm not doing it myself. It won't work if I don't walk the walk. I confer with other people who can support me and who can help me think and talk through my work. I look at it as the domino effect, and it comes full circle. I get support and then I'm able to support others. I have to be accountable so that I can be a leader.

It's not my program. It's our program. And they're all a part of it.

They're a part of every single piece of it, and it's funny because I'm supposed to take a sabbatical, and I've taught just about everyone how to do my job. I have no concerns about someone trying to take my job. I think it builds trust if they know what I'm doing. Advocates know that there's the good, the bad, and the ugly in this work. The good is when your heart wants to help; the bad is when you don't feel like the system is on your side; and the ugly is the hoops you have to jump through to keep things running. If advocates are aware of all the aspects of the job, then they are more inclined to be invested in the results at the end. If I treat them like I'm superior to them and act like I have all the answers, then I lose that trust and they lose respect for their job and me. How do I do this? I include them when decisions need to be made. I want them to be creative in their work; I want them to reach out and network with others, join agency committees, or go to outside trainings. I want them to do more than just come to work.

When we need to hire a new staff person, they take turns on the hiring committee with me so they can understand what that process is like. I want their support with bringing on a new staff person. I try to create a space where everyone is included. There's no us and them. I think creating that space of safety helps cut down on the impact of trauma exposure. When something is about to go down, we can deal with the trauma that is coming in the front door. You can deal with the impact that that woman's story is going to have on you because of the way we support one another.

I think I'm here because I have figured out how to do the job and also to be of support to others. I'm driven to help others do this work and be successful at it. By successful, I mean doing it and being healthy. Because really, I don't see the end of domestic violence coming anytime soon, so to me, being successful is being able to do it while you're still taking care of yourself. It matters because people who are in need are coming to us for services, and we have to be ready for whatever they're about to say, and I think the healthier we are, the better we are able to provide supportive services. If a woman comes in and says, "I've been held in my house and I wasn't able to leave, and my child was sexually abused and I don't know what to do," I know at this point that this woman, one, needs to talk; two, needs some counseling; three, needs help to attend to her child. I'm able to give her the appropriate support and not just refer her to another office because she's not just a number to me. It's sad to see advocates who are burned out and will treat women like a number.

    The advocates care a great deal about the children that come in with the women. They will go that extra, extra, extra mile for a child. You're not only looking at a woman who's been traumatized, you're looking at a child who has also suffered a traumatic situation. I think it's amazing when they can support both groups of people.

I think this is what I'm here to do. I don't think it's an accident. I'm here for a reason. I have an ability to support others who support others, and why not? Isn't that what the whole world needs? People want to have connection and support. That's what we all need. So if I can give in this small way, that means a lot ... to me.

CHAPTER SIX

Coming into the Present Moment

> Abandon any hope of fruition. The key instruction is to stay in the present. Don't get caught up in hopes of what you'll achieve and how good your situation will be some day in the future. What you do right now is what matters.
>
> Pema Chödrön, Tibetan Buddhist nun and resident teacher of Gampo Abbey, Nova Scotia

As I turned toward trauma stewardship, I sought input and direction from every wise person and every loving tradition I could find. Whether in a dharma talk, pipe circle, temazcal, or midrash, or in the teachings and biographies of Nelson Mandela, Pema Chödrön, Desmond Tutu, Wangari Maathai, Thich Nhat Hanh, Viktor Frankl, and others, I looked for the specific ways that people maintained clarity and wisdom in the face of suffering. Whether the suffering originated in the polluting of a country's water supply or in the horrors of apartheid, the method was similar. The ancient traditions and the contemporary teachers I studied consistently valued one thing in particular: being awake, present, and aware in this moment.

As I studied and practiced, I became interested in the recurrence of this idea. While it is an understatement to say that the cultural, spiritual, and religious traditions I explored have many differences, the wisdom of present awareness draws them together. Each tradition draws on centuries of distinct experience, but at the core of their collective wisdom is an invitation to live your life from the here and now, not in an anticipated future or a ruminated past.

There are a number of reasons why being in the present moment is helpful in trauma stewardship. One is that until we slow down enough to honestly feel how we are doing, we can't assess our current state and what we need. As the American actress, playwright, and screenwriter Mae West said, "When in doubt, take a bath." When we keep ourselves numbed out on adrenaline or overworking or cynicism, we don't have an accurate internal gauge of ourselves and our needs. (Figure 6.1)

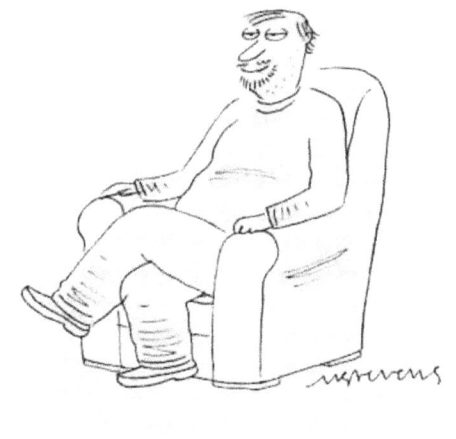

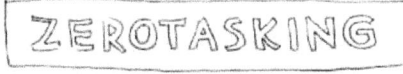

Figure 6.1

According to Peter Levine, what we need to do is to attune to our "felt sense." The felt sense is what tells you where you are and how you feel, moment by moment. While it is subtle and we often take it for granted, it is an extremely powerful first step to "trust your gut." Levine states, "Nature has not forgotten us, we have forgotten it. A traumatized person's nervous system is not damaged; it is frozen in a kind of suspended animation. Rediscovering the felt sense will bring warmth and vitality to our experiences…. We have built-in mechanisms for responding to and moving towards natural resolution of trauma."

Hyperintellectualism occurs when we seek to abandon the felt sense altogether. We may attempt to move out of our bodies, hearts, and spirits to live only in our heads. In humans, part of the left cortex in our brains is programmed to try to make meaning of our experiences. Thus, we can see how when humans become profoundly overwhelmed or confused, a natural place to take refuge is in our rationalizing minds and in our left brain. There, the brain is working double-time to arrange our experiences into some sort of rational, manageable order—even if this order is wholly disconnected from our right hemisphere's experience of the felt sense. One thing we want to explore, however, is how we can bring our felt sense and our sense of meaning together—in other words, how we can reconcile the two distinct impressions to create an "integrated state," as Daniel Siegel refers to it in his work on the neurobiology of mindfulness.

Charles Newcomb, an engineer and scientist who works with renewable energy assets (solar panels, wind turbines) all over the world, describes the disconnect that happens for him when he gets overly heady in trying to cope with what he sees. "I fall back into this rational mind that says, 'If we all die because of global warming, it'll be fine.' Because I see a tremendous lack of discipline in our species—the urgency of greed is so much more vital than the sensibility of sustainability, and I don't have a lot of faith. I think sometimes we need that perfect plague to wake us up and release our footprint from this earth. But then I think of one of my children dying from the avian flu. I think about who would be the first to die, and I realize I can't think that way anymore."

A veterinarian and scientist working on conservation medicine for endangered species and animal welfare in Asia talks about trying to mitigate the impact of her work by staying in her head: "I reconcile what I see through an intellectualization of the biology and behavior of humans and the determinism of the physical universe. Not that I have been able to use this rationalization to lessen my grief and anger, try as I do. One simply cannot afford to let up on the very firm grip that one must maintain on one's emotions. At least, that is the way it is for me."

As we deepen our ability to make contact with our inner selves, we slowly build our capacity for self-diagnosis and self-healing. Dr. Liu Dong is a master of qigong, an ancient Chinese healing art based on Taoist principles. His tradition teaches that the more we know what is going on externally in the world, the less we know what is going on internally in ourselves. Like other Taoists, Dr. Liu believes that we all hold a piece of the universal spirit. As we live our lives and become attached to the outside world, this light within—which some traditions call the divine, some call *yuan shen,* some call self-awareness—becomes clouded over.

By coming into the present moment and bringing our awareness within us, we can self-purify and self-transform.

These Chinese teachings state that self-healing and early diagnosis of personal ailments comes out of quieting our external attachments and channeling all our energy into one intention—an act of focus that leads us to the qigong state, which we hope eventually to experience in every moment. The qigong state can happen only in the now. It puts us in touch with our divine, brilliant nature. When we are in it, we receive energy from the universe instead of letting it be drained from us. While Chinese medicine acknowledges it is human nature to be externally focused, Dr. Liu grew up being told, "Study, but not too much. Think, but not too much."

These beliefs are reflected in other traditions around the world. Science is beginning to reflect what sages, shamans, and healers have known for centuries. Brain wave testing shows that many healers, from Native American medicine men and women performing rituals to meditating Buddhist monks and nuns, reach a state in which their brains are producing delta waves, the same type of brain waves that newborns produce day-to-day. As Kenneth Cohen writes in his book *The Way of Qigong,*

> The slowest is delta (.5-4 Hz), prevalent during infancy or, in adults, during deep sleep. Healers sometimes produce delta while awake, a graphic example of connecting with the wisdom of childhood and accessing the deepest levels of consciousness.... The quickest brain waves, beta (13-26 Hz or higher), characterize adult waking consciousness most of the time.... The beta predominant state is euphemistically called 'awareness,' but is most prevalent during states of free floating anxiety, when the mind is restless, according to energy medicine researcher, the late Ed Wilson, M.D. It is likely that a large percentage of the adult U.S. population is chronically stuck in beta while awake. We tend to 'think about' rather than experience silently. Thinking is a useful and essential means of interpreting

experience, but it is pathological if it dominates consciousness.

This may, in part, be why parents of newborns often don't lay their infants down in a bed once they are asleep, even though they themselves are extremely sleep deprived. Holding a sleeping baby, they may feel an essential life energy that, for many of us, can be experienced only at the hands of healers.

When we are able to make ourselves as still within as an untouched mountain lake, we have an exquisite reflection of all that is in and around us. When ripples do arise, we can recognize their source, whether it is the rain or the wind or the fish jumping. Without the stillness, all we know is that the waters are tumultuous, and we may want to do anything possible to escape the feeling of unease. (Figure 6.2)

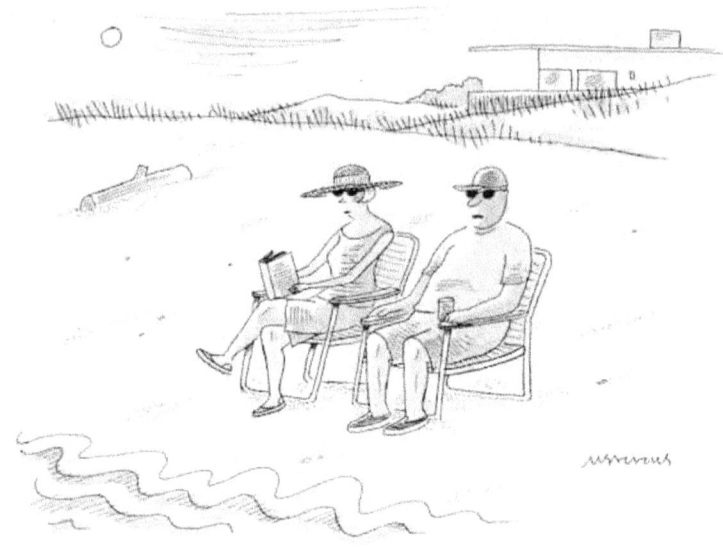

Figure 6.2: "I can't stop thinking about all those available parking spaces back on West Eighty-fifth Street."

Many of us who work in helping professions are used to operating at a sprint, so coming into the present moment may feel like a powerful contradiction. Nevertheless, it is difficult to appreciate our lives when we are not paying attention to them in a conscious way. As one child support worker told me, "I feel like I've missed out on my whole life."

There are innumerable ways to return to stillness, including such centering acts as breathing, meditation, mindful movement, and prayer. Any of these can be a saving grace, and they are all free and portable. It is worth noting, however, that the challenges of getting to a place where we can come into the present moment and experience inner stillness may be considerable. The difficulties aren't only internal but external. Modern culture, in its many manifestations around the globe, has rejected many of the ancient traditions that value coming into the present moment. The consumerist ethos that took such a firm hold in the 20th century urges us to strive for more (money, clothes, cars, houses, objects). As we move deeper into the information age, the media industry wants us to feel left out if we're not literally plugged into the latest music, movie, commercial, or game. With all these pressures, it's no wonder that few of us find time to connect with ourselves.

Being present is real work. Meditation and yoga are referred to as practices for a reason—they require repetition and commitment to a process. In one workshop, Dr. Liu Dong said of qigong, "The first half-hour or so of any practice session is usually just about pain." Similarly, a friend told me about his visit to a Burmese monastery where he had hoped to study for three weeks. Hearing of this proposed time frame, a monk said, "It won't be worth it for you. Generally the first five months here are full of suffering, and after that you begin to reap the benefits."

> One step, one foot in front of the other: That's how we're going to do it.
> Community activist in New Orleans, post-Hurricane Katrina

Still, while this practice is not for the faint of heart, it should not be seen as inaccessible. You are fully capable of becoming present. Sometimes it is very hard and sometimes it is very simple, but you must be willing to introduce some new habits as a counterpoint to your old familiar ways. For example, during a recent vacation with my family, I was struck by how entrenched my patterns of thinking were. I was thousands of miles away from the 11 children who attend school at my home each day and all my other at-home responsibilities, but it took nothing for me to transfer my sense of worry and alertness to conditions on the beach. Was it low tide or high tide? Would those clouds eventually produce rain? How were the surfing conditions? It was absurd, as none of these things *really* mattered at all. But I was amused by how diligently my mind was working, and in its habitual way—the surroundings had changed dramatically, but my thoughts maintained the vigilant status quo. Once I came into the present moment enough to notice my thoughts, I was able to stop the pattern. I returned my awareness to my family and the sensations of air and sand.

PROFILE CHERI MAPLES

MADISON, WISCONSIN
CURRENTLY: Outgoing assistant attorney general for Wisconsin; criminal justice consultant.

FORMERLY: Head of probation and parole for the State of Wisconsin; administrator for the Division of Community Corrections; police officer; director of the

Wisconsin Coalition of Domestic Violence; community education specialist for a domestic violence shelter; Federal Neighborhood Housing Project community organizer.

I had been the first director of the Wisconsin Coalition Against Domestic Violence. Then I went to get a Ph.D. and hated it. During that time, I was with my partner for 10 years, and together we had two children and three stepchildren. I was working as a teacher's assistant in women's studies, and I was not making enough money to support a family with five kids, so I dropped out of the Ph.D. program in the last semester. There was a very progressive police chief at the time, and so I joined the police department and went on to have a 20-year career there. I served as an officer, sergeant, lieutenant, and captain.

In 1991, seven years into my job (I was a sergeant at the time), I had herniated a disc on the job and went to a chiropractor for a while. It was in her waiting room that I read an article about Thich Nhat Hanh, or Thây, as his students call him. I had to take some time off because of the injury, and I went to my first Thich Nhat Hanh retreat out of curiosity. It was in Illinois and it was pretty small, and I went to a presentation of the five mindfulness trainings.

I was very used to people making assumptions about me because I was a cop, and so I was a little bit defensive. During these mindfulness trainings there's an opportunity to take a vow to follow these teachings, and one is about being determined not to kill and not to let others kill. I said, "I can't take this because I'm a cop," and Sister Chan Khong, one of the original members of the Order of Interbeing, pulled me aside and said, "Who else would we want to carry a gun besides someone who would do it mindfully?" That first retreat was a start to what changed my life. I got a taste of what mindfulness is about and what slowing down and being in the present means.

When I came back to work after that, it was really interesting, because I was so present that it felt like everyone was changing, and I realized it was the energy I was putting out. That is what got me interested, this realization that others were changing all around me, in part as a result of how I had changed. I went through two relationships, one a 10-year and one a 13-year. This is not unusual for cops. Because of what I faced when I came in as a woman and an out lesbian, I had my levels of anger about that, and from growing up in my family, I had a lot of edges to work on. I got sober shortly before finding Thây. That was my initial road to spirituality, and I started to realize that policing was full of effects that took their toll over time.

As the captain of personnel and training, I kept going to retreats and doing meditation and reading, and I realized we weren't losing people physically. We had great hiring practices, we kept people safe, but I saw people change before my eyes. I realized we were losing people emotionally because of secondary trauma. There is the incredible adrenaline rush you get at work, and then you go home and the things that make you a good police officer don't make you a good partner, and so there's this crash when you get home and people shut down.

At work you feel on top of the world with adrenaline, and you're above the normal risk level that people experience, and a lot of people have this experience of being overdriven and multitasking all the time. You go to work, you get high, then you come home and crash, and you keep repeating this, and the bottom of that cycle feels like depression, and then I think people find dysfunctional ways to deal. You associate that low end of the cycle with your family and your friends, because you don't understand it. You don't understand completely what is going on.

I began to do trainings on this, and I learned to translate the language from my spiritual journey into what law enforcement would understand, and so I called it health and wellness and ethics and diversity training. I insisted that we incorporate ethics into our curriculum. We worked on the unspoken agreements and socialization that go on in law enforcement culture that's stronger than anything on paper and amounts to more. I did these trainings for law enforcement, judges, and attorneys. Also while I was at the police department, I did optional mindfulness trainings for police officers. I tried to change the existing agreements we had in this law enforcement culture, and I think I had some success at that.

I got ordained by Thich Nhat Hanh in Plum Village, France, in 2002, and then in 2003 I brought Thây here with the help of my sangha and the international sangha to do a retreat for criminal justice and helping professionals. I got a lot of criticism and some hate mail, and I got called to the city attorney's office to explain myself, and there were times that I was wondering if this was worthwhile. It started taking such a personal and emotional toll. I just had to keep asking myself during that time, "What are your intentions?" The training ended up being really good, and I think it was very transformational for people who went there. The officers provided a session from their hearts for everyone there on the last night that was very powerful. It was amazing for these police officers to see that they could share themselves emotionally with others and talk about what it was like to be a police officer and what the toll was like, including others' perceptions of them.

I came back and I ran for chief of police, and I was one of two finalists and I had a lot internal support. I was prepared for either result, and I believed that if the conditions were right, I would get it, and if not, I wouldn't. I really didn't enjoy the whole process and the public figure aspect of it. It was very exhausting and a lot of responsibility, and that still continues to a certain extent. I did not get that job, and after I left the police department, I was recruited to be the head of probation and parole for the State of Wisconsin. I had a very good experience there, although it was very overwhelming, but I did a lot with issues of race, ethics, and health and wellness.

I got to be a part of starting what I think is the most creative public safety project while I was there. It's the Dane County Time Bank (danecountytimebank.org), which created a bartering system that helped equalize class and access to resources. For example, we did a prevention project for kids who are being arrested and having their first contact with cops. The cops refer them to youth court, where they face a jury of their peers, and if they complete the sentence, they get time dollars. We also started a reintegration program for people leaving prison. I remain the president of the board. I ultimately got frustrated with my work at that time, because it was a governor-appointed job and very demanding, and even though my son was away at school, it was still overwhelming. I understood that it was about protecting the governor from the next Willie Horton, so I left, but I stayed on doing consulting.

I was then recruited by the attorney general, and I'm currently an assistant attorney general. She promised me any projects, any hours, and I have had a great run here doing a combination of active community organizing projects as well as being able to train people at the Department of Justice in mindfulness under the health and wellness title. I also had an opportunity to work with a statewide coalition to expand the project that involves making community policing stronger. I put the mindfulness trainings into language they can understand—for example, verbal judo instead of nonviolent communication. You have to get credibility in your profession, and now I've worked in about all parts of the criminal justice system, and so I have a lot of contacts and I've earned credibility. I'm not just some wacko New Age person, and they get that I understand their job. I feel really good about how this has come into the criminal justice system. I feel blessed with what the practice has brought and continues to bring to my life.

I've always worked with issues of social justice, and since I've started down this path of mindfulness, I do my work very differently, and it's much more effective. I firmly believe that the most important part of this work is the work we do on ourselves, and then it becomes automatic, being able to incorporate all the teachings. It's like when you look at Thây; it's not what he says, it's the way he moves. The way he moves is a dharma talk. It's just being around him. And I love it that he encourages people to go back to their root traditions, so that this way of being in the world is accessible to anyone.

When I think about the toll my work has had on me, one of the things that is interesting about mindfulness practice is that we're really encouraged not to consume violence. Well, police officers are forced to consume violence on a daily basis. We're forced to face the situations that you don't want to hear about. You're the one who goes to where there are brains all over the scene after a car accident, and you know all the sad stories and the suffering that goes on behind closed doors, and to deal with that kind of secondary trauma, even though it's not necessarily apparent to you at the time, it's there.

And there is this whole machismo socialization of "Are you tough enough to take care of yourself and others, and do it without being impacted?" It's hard, too, because there's a job to be done, so you have to close down some to do the job or you won't be able to do it. I realize that before I started this practice, however, I was no longer doing my job with any heart. And at some point you are not effective at your job anymore, because of your lack of understanding with what you're facing and what you're feeling.

I think to take care of yourself involves three things. First, you need to understand the cycle and what's happening and see it for what it is. Second, it is important not to have all your best friends as police officers. There's an us-versus-them mentality of "Only I and my coworkers understand this and no one else will understand," and so I make sure to limit my contact with other police officers outside of work. I never had a partner who was a police officer. I learned and developed an understanding that the command presence required to take charge and develop good interview and interrogation skills at work aren't the things that lead to you being a good partner in intimate relationships. You have to sort that out.

Someone has to do this job, and I have a lot of respect for police officers, and I love Wisconsin statutes because they call us peace officers. I think it's a very noble profession, and it's a very difficult profession. You don't want to have contact with a police officer, because if you do, it means something is wrong. It's really hard to get any support from the general public to do your job.

Third, to take care of myself, I've developed a daily practice; I have a sangha, and I think Thây's idea that you need a community to support you is extremely important. I have a partner who is committed to the same spiritual values, and I have a community of people who I surround myself with and who are extremely supportive of this work, and they see that this takes courage. I have my own support system that will help me further the values and help me understand the ways that I'm blind and ways I've been co-opted, so I stay honest.

I don't know what's next, but it will be something. I've always had great stages put in front of me, great places from which I can work. You try to do the next right thing in front of you, and the rest takes care of itself.

There was a time in my life when I didn't do that, and I didn't understand that coming from an emotional place is a whole different world than coming from an intellectual place.

I consider myself a beginner in this. The thing that I love about Thây's understanding about police officers is that he understands there's a need for both gentle compassion and fierce compassion. If you do both with the right intention in your heart, and not out of a place of anger, you get a lot further. And that's the big difference. From what place do you do your work? What's in your heart and how do you approach your work? You must make peace in the space of your own heart before you can take this stuff any further.

PART FOUR

FINDING YOUR WAY TO TRAUMA STEWARDSHIP

CHAPTER SEVEN

Following the Five Directions

As you begin your journey, remember that you are not alone. Nearly every spiritual tradition has created stories or texts to guide the way. Any one of these might help you to arrive at answers that will allow you to benefit yourself and others to the fullest extent. For this book, I have created the Five Directions as a navigational tool. It is our compass: It will help us to continuously assess how we are doing and what we need.

In developing the Five Directions, I have drawn upon a vision of the world that was common to many early cultures in Asia, the Americas, and even in Europe. In addition to the four cardinal directions—north, east, south, and west—the ancients envisioned a fifth direction. This was sometimes seen as the core element that linked Earth to both the heavens and the underworld. It has been variously described as "the center," "here," or the "spiritual direction."

The ancients understood this fifth direction to be integrally connected to the other four. In the modern world, we often think of north, east, south, and west as little more than the letters at the ends of arrows pointing our way across the earth's terrain. To the earlier peoples, of course, each of the directions was linked to natural phenomena—and therefore with colors, materials, and seasons, as well as with their metaphorical qualities. East, for example, is the direction of dawn. To the Chinese, east was often associated with springtime, the colors green and blue, and wood; to the Cherokee nation, on the other hand, east was associated with the color red, reawakening from winter, and new life.

From such descriptions, it is easy to understand how the individual points of the compass came to be closely associated with different aspects of spiritual experience. In Native American traditions in particular, the human journey through life is often described in terms of the interplay of five directions. Each of us travels to the symbolic destinations represented by the four cardinal directions at some point in our lives; every journey leads us both away from our center and back toward it.

As by now you will recognize, this model very closely parallels the process by which we can build our capacity for trauma stewardship. For our purposes, the fifth direction is our own interconnected human core—our centered self. Our experiences as we tread each new path will vary depending on who we are as individuals, but we also open ourselves up to the possibility that we can learn from these experiences and they may change us.

So when we have our next encounter, we may approach the world differently than we did before. Our center is our guide, and yet if we are living fully, that center will be ever-evolving.

As we do our work, we continually seek strength by finding our center in the present moment. At the same time, we strive to enhance our self-knowledge by focusing consciously and concretely on the basic elements of our lives. The things we learn at the four outlying points of our compass of trauma stewardship will become the tools we can use to build a daily practice of centering ourselves. As we deepen our connection with our center, we tap into our innate qualities of wisdom, free will, compassion, and balance.

The Five Directions offer a description of the world and a set of instructions for making our way through it. They guide a process through which we can create and maintain our well-being, even during the most turbulent times. Honoring traditions from around the globe, we allow each of these directions to assist us in returning to the place where our greatest hope for understanding, peace, health, fulfillment, and joy exists: within ourselves.

You may use the Five Directions in several ways. As you begin, you may wish to focus on the points of our compass only as I have already described them: inquiry, focus, compassion, balance, and centering. In time, however, you may find it helpful to think about the Five Directions using other types of imagery. I will begin the discussion of each direction by briefly invoking some of the colors and elements that are typically associated with that direction. Each of us will take a different path to reach our center. For some of us, it may be more effective to summon the feelings of sustenance that come with the earth, which is associated with the south, than to think rationally about community and compassion. For others, the opposite may be true. The additional characterizations of each direction are intended to expand your options.

As you can see from the illustration on the inside back cover, each direction is unique, yet they fit together to form a vibrant whole. Simply looking at this image may provide a quick visual reminder of what's important as you orient yourself from day to day. Try taking a few minutes to meditate on the directions, whether you are commuting to or from work, going about your business, or lying in bed at night. This is one way to create a daily mindfulness practice. Of course, you can use the Five Directions as inspiration for rituals of your own.

By moving among the directions and their elements, we are able to create, and most important, maintain, a daily practice through which we become centered. When we are centered, we are in the fifth direction. There will be times in our lives and our work when the water turns into a tidal wave, the fire into an inferno, the earth into quicksand, and the air into a tornado. We may feel overwhelmed, bombarded, off our game, and at a loss, sometimes several times each day. The Five Directions can guide us to regain calm—to once again remember who we are, where we're headed, and what we need. Being centered allows us to occupy a constant oasis of wisdom, perspective, and integrity, regardless of how out of control everything and everyone around us seems. As we build our personal practice, we can approach our circumstances proactively rather than reactively. With sustained effort, we can maintain the inner resources we need to care for ourselves and to care for others and the planet. This ability is the foundation of trauma stewardship.

In the chapters ahead, I will make various suggestions for building your practice. I offer the Five Directions to those who welcome guidance as they enter a new path. Should you be someone who prefers to keep your mind free as you explore, read on with confidence that your daily practice will evolve in its own unique way.

CHAPTER EIGHT

NORTH • Creating Space for Inquiry

We begin our journey in the north, where we call upon the courage and wisdom of the water element. We do this by coming into the present moment—by stopping our mind's chatter and simply noticing what is around us. We try to create a sense of spaciousness—a horizon as vast as the one we see when looking out across the ocean. From this expansive vantage point, we will ask ourselves two critical questions: "Why am I doing what I'm doing?" and "Is this working for me?" (In order to answer these questions, we will also examine the concept of trauma mastery.) *Just as all known forms of life depend on water, the quality of our livelihood depends on understanding our intention in regard to our work.*

Why Am I Doing What I'm Doing?

I once saw Jorge Alvarado, a Coahuiltec pipe carrier and Lakota Sun Dancer, work with a woman in a healing Ceremony. He told her, "You are the kind of person who is going to have to ask yourself every day, 'Who am I and what am I doing here?'" On some level, these are questions for each of us to answer. Mindfulness begins with being alert to our sensations in the present moment, and it extends to a larger awareness of what we are doing in our lives. In my experience, however, it is difficult to be fully aware of what we are doing if we are oblivious to what motivates us to do it. Few things are as powerful as knowing why we're doing what we're doing. As the 19th-century Prussian philosopher Friedrich Nietzsche said, "He who has a why to live for can bear with almost any how."

When we apply this kind of inquiry to our work, it gives us a framework for understanding our intentions, motivations, and hopes. Why have we chosen to make the effort toward helping or healing such a prominent part of our lives?

I encourage people to be honest with themselves about why they are currently engaged in their work. Start with the simplest of questions and see where they lead you. What gets you on the bus in the morning? What keeps you showing up at the community meetings? Perhaps it's because you have an important contribution to bring to your field, or perhaps it's because you don't know where your résumé is on your hard drive. Maybe you desperately need the health insurance, or maybe you're terrified of change. Maybe you're hoping to achieve trauma mastery, which we will discuss later in this chapter. Regardless of the answer, checking in with yourself about why you're doing what you're doing can make all the difference in understanding that you have a choice.

> Could this be why I'm doing this work? Because my people are so often the ones being put away in the prison complexes? There's a story in my family of my

grandmother, who was not able to get out of her rocking chair, but she pistol-whipped a white policeman with a pistol she kept with her, because he came to arrest my uncle for a crime. My uncle had been home the whole day washing clothes by hand at the side of the house. He'd been there all day, but this policeman came to take him, and my grandma beat the officer until he left. It's always stayed with me, that story. It's always been in my mind.

John Brookins, former Black Panther; prison reentry specialist, Village of Hope; director of men's inistry, Freedom Church, Seattle, Washington

Being clear each day about "Why am I doing this work?" requires opportunities for reflection. As we discussed in chapter 2, some organizations adapt to the crises they address in their work by adopting a crisis mode in their organizational structures. Such organizations may have created working cultures that penalize reflection and reward plugging along. You may have to make a commitment to persevere with reflection even in the face of opposition or a lack of understanding from your organization and colleagues.

If you start to waver, remind yourself that reflection is a powerful antidote to the helplessness we may feel as a result of trauma exposure. Amid the trials and tribulations of our work, it is possible to lose sight of why we're doing what we're doing. When we carve out the time to contemplate our intentions, we renew our connection to the needs and desires that have shaped our experience. We remember that we can take action to alter the course of our lives. This will help us to alleviate the sensation of being tossed around in the waves of uncontrollable and overwhelming events. (Figure 8.1)

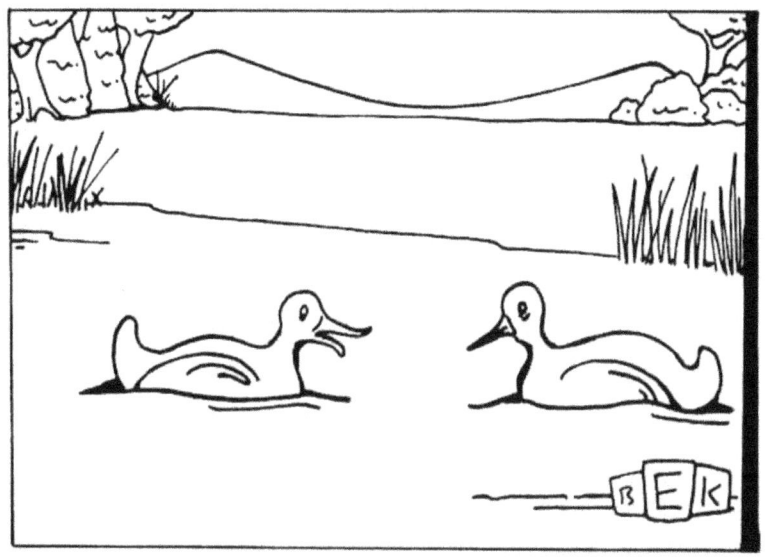

Figure 8.1: "Maybe you should ask yourself why you're inviting all this duck hunting into your life right now."

TRY THIS

1. Before starting your workday, take a moment to literally stop in your tracks and ask yourself, "Why am I doing what I am doing?" After you hear your answer, remind yourself, gently, that you are making a choice to do this work. Take a deep breath; breathe in both the responsibility and the freedom in this acknowledgment.

2. Regularly consult with someone about why you are doing what you are doing. Choose a trustworthy, supportive, wise person. Ask this person to listen attentively and provide you with feedback. It is critical to not be isolated in our work.

3. Regularly write down why you are doing what you're doing, what your intention is. Keep it somewhere. When you feel yourself going astray, return from that client consult, staff meeting, or board retreat and find your written intention. Remind yourself what it is about for you, and what it is definitely not about.

PROFILE THE NORTHWEST IMMIGRANT RIGHTS PROJECT

The Northwest Immigrant Rights Project (NWIRP) is an organization that has worked for over 25 years to advance the legal rights and dignity of low-income immigrants in Washington State by pursuing and preserving their legal status through legal representation, education, and public policy. NWIRP serves all nationalities, including low-income immigrants from Latin America, Asia, the Middle East, Eastern and Western Europe, and Africa. When I worked with NWIRP on issues of trauma stewardship in the 1990s, its culture seemed special and wonderful. The tremendous dedication of the workers and unending compassion they held for their clients was palpable every single time I went there. It was, and remains, a very special place.

For as long as it has existed, NWIRP has handled heart-wrenching and urgent cases, many of which literally involve life and death. By the mid-1990s, however, it was no longer able to handle the full volume of calls. The attorneys were juggling so many court actions that they began to fear they'd botch some client's case and be sued for malpractice. At the end of their rope, they instructed the intake staff to start turning less needy clients away.

Donna Lewen, who worked with NWIRP as the coordinator of the domestic violence unit for seven years, shares, "When I picture that decision, I remember the look in the eyes of the frontline staff, who were the ones to take the calls and hear horrendous story after horrendous story about people who were facing death and desperately needed legal help. They would have to say, 'I'm sorry, we can't take any more cases.' And where could you send them? There was nowhere else to send most of them. It was overwhelming for the intake staff to have to say this to people." The workers began to disintegrate under the burden.

The situation became untenable, and after much input from the staff, NWIRP's executive director at the time, Vicky Stifter, made an exceptionally difficult decision: NWIRP would shut down its intake entirely. Until they could resolve the problems, they would not accept any new clients. It was an effort to "save a sinking ship," Stifter recalls. "We were taking on more than we could handle, and we were all going down."

Stifter felt it was her responsibility as executive director to step in and ease the crisis for her staff.

It was easier for me to do it from a far than it would have been for an individual who had to hear the stories directly. When individuals in an organization are left on their own to make limits, and they're the ones who are confronting the person in trauma, face to face and over and over again, it's impossible for them. It's incumbent on the organization to make these decisions.

The hope was that [closing intake] would allow folks to be more solid individually and collectively and to feel some of that incredible stress diminish. I wanted to protect people from their exposure to trauma as an organization. It was an incredibly difficult decision to make, and when you see these people coming to you in need, it's heart-wrenching to not respond. But we all knew [that keeping intake open] wasn't going to take us anywhere good, and even if we did take on more cases, we still weren't going to meet the need out there. We needed to be as strategic and healthy about it as possible.

There was significant internal conflict before this decision was made. The frontline staff found it hard to contain the helplessness they felt; it was easier to be enraged and blame others on staff for not doing everything they could. For their part, the attorneys knew they could no longer responsibly manage their caseload in the current state of the organization. Yet some of them wanted to blame intake—if intake had been screening clients at an optimal level, they speculated, maybe the closing could have been averted.

Lewen recalls, "It was unclear how long we were going to stay closed, and the longer the closure was extended, the more demoralizing it felt to me. You're still so underwater and trying to get your bearings. The organization is far over capacity, so everyone's working bad hours, and that whittles away at you. You make it a little more manageable, and yet you're still exhausted and still recovering, and now you're leaving at 6p.m. instead of 7p.m. It was amazing to realize that we were still so busy and we weren't even accepting new cases. How were we ever doing it before, and how were we ever going to do it again?"

She continues, "We started working on a plan based on the reality that we could not do everything. We started asking ourselves, 'How are we going to do what we do as well as we can? How are we going to protect those whose job it is to turn people away?' I remember thinking, 'Let's not fancy ourselves as the only place that can assist these people.'" Stifter echoes this. "We're called to do something somewhere, but it's self-aggrandizement to feel like I have to take it all on and take care of everyone," she says. "So part of it is the humility of realizing this is my piece, and I want to tend to this piece the best I can, but I'm not in charge of the whole garden."

In time, NWIRP would make a number of changes to streamline its operation. It hired an outside consultant to assist the staff in coming up with a long-term plan. It started orienting clients in groups rather than one on one, created more print materials, and limited the hours and days of intake. It also developed a phone system for providing initial information to potential clients. Rather than asking the intake staff to redirect clients in person, NWIRP began stating its policy via an automated voice message. Lewen recounts, "We asked ourselves, 'Is it a meaningful use of resources to have a live person on the phone turning people away? Is it ethical not to have a live person doing this?'"

The reality of closing intake was hard. Some community leaders and organizations were supportive, while others were judgmental and even disgusted. Lewen wrestled with the criticism but also remembers thinking,

"We are part of a much larger and troubled judicial system. Why am I feeling personally responsible for our foreign policy?"

Jonathan Moore, a paralegal who was an accredited representative at NWIRP for 16 years, was told that the closure had harmed NWIRP's reputation as an agency. "It was very demoralizing to think that this could be perceived as undermining the very heart of our work for social justice," he recalls. "For those who had the direct contact with the public every single day, the intake workers, it was very harsh to experience people denouncing you." Stifter too describes how awful it was to deal with community members who could not understand NWIRP's intentions. The closure was "not widely accepted. I don't hold it out as the best strategy, but I do think that figuring out how to not get overloaded is critical, and when you can't, then sometimes the only response is to stop entirely."

While the decision to close intake was hard, Lewen says, "things were meaningfully different as a result. I just remember feeling a sense of some relief and some quiet. There's a feeling of futility when you're up against as much as we had been. There's this constant clamor in your head, which is filled with the desire to help others and the painful knowledge of what you can't do, and it never goes away. During that time, we were still working like crazy, but now we could focus less fleetingly on each person. You're not combat-lawyering anymore. You're not internalizing crises all the time. We had the space and sanity to reflect on what we were doing instead of what we weren't getting done. I think it helped reduce the clamor in our minds. And still, it always felt urgent to open back up our intake. Even if closing intake felt like the responsible thing to do, nobody felt OK about it."

Moore says, "I remember when you had to do a removal case from the beginning to the end of the hearing. It's pretty labor intensive and you really want to do a good job.

You're doing it all on your own, and so there's this tension between doing the cases you have really well and doing more cases, and of course your loyalty is to the people you're actually representing. You can't prioritize an obligation on a case you haven't taken, but still you think about it. You want to document everything on your cases and maybe you're doing too much, but you never know. You have to judge when what you've done is enough and when you could take on more. And that's hard."

Another NWIRP staffer revealed how few options people felt they had for slowing down before the closing. She herself felt that "the only legitimate justification for withdrawing my energy at all was to have a baby. I remember thinking that was the only way I'd be able to stop doing what I was doing. Fortunately, I also wanted a baby, but isn't that disturbing?" She knew she wanted her work life to be different. "When we're doing social justice work, we are really wanting everyone to live better, not as bad as the worst surviving person. If we really understood what it is like to live in such impoverished conditions, then we wouldn't be glamorizing it like we do on some level through our work environments."

Moore remembers, "We were always trying to reinvent how we did intake. Sometimes it seemed like we were just moving around the problem, but there was always a lot of discussion in the organization and I think that really helped." Stifter says, "'Trauma exposure response' wasn't in my vocabulary at that time, but I wish it had been. I think I would have been more effective if I had known exactly what individuals were facing, if I had known there were things to look for, and that it has a name." Beginning with the closing of intake, NWIRP moved in the direction of more moderation. Once moderation was adopted as an organizational strategy, Stifter says, "it seeped through, and when folks came into that culture anew, they had different expectations."

She describes her evolution toward achieving balance in her life. "I had lost my own personal life. I had lost a lot of small things along the way. A big turning point was having children and realizing that this isn't going to work, and the cost is too great. Some of the best things I've done have resulted from a focus of, I'm going to do this and say 'no' to these 12 things, and that is OK. I've seen how fruitful that can be. When I was the executive director of NWIRP, I would go swimming three afternoons a week at the YMCA, and people would remark on this. They didn't understand how I could take the time away. I'd tell them, 'I just walk out the front door. That's all it takes.' I'd be gone an hour. I'd just go swimming and know that it was OK. All my work was there when I got back. And I was better for having gone."

Vicky Stifter is now a pastor at a church in Hood River, Oregon, and we ended our conversation just in time: "Come hell or high water, I've made

> *a commitment to go to this yoga class every Tuesday, so I have to go now."*

Is Trauma Mastery a Factor for Me?

> I miss my trauma.
> Trauma survivor

As we consider why we're doing what we're doing, it may be useful to check in with ourselves about the presence of trauma mastery in our lives. Trauma mastery addresses one way of coping with trauma. For many survivors of trauma, our lack of control over a traumatic incident is one of the most terrifying and unnerving things about it. How much anxiety this causes us will vary from person to person, depending on how much control we feel like we have in life generally. Our philosophy or spirituality or religion may tell us to have faith in a higher power—but still, one of the hardest things about trauma is this feeling of not being in control.

What humans often do to reconcile this lack of control is to create and re-create situations as similar to the traumatic incident as possible. We seek to turn a traumatic situation in which we once felt powerless into a new situation where we feel competent and in charge. We tell ourselves that this time there will be a different outcome. Or so we hope. This is a sophisticated coping mechanism, and by and large it is done unconsciously. If we are conscious that we are seeking trauma mastery, and if we navigate with insight, mindfulness, and honesty, this mechanism may contribute to our healing. More often, though, our attempts at trauma mastery lack awareness and intention. We act reflexively, attempting to salvage some sense of control. We can end up reinforcing feelings of being overwhelmed or lacking power—at its extreme, unconscious trauma mastery may even increase our risk of physical harm or exposure to dangerous situations. This is obviously to our detriment, and the cycle of attempting to master the trauma is likely to start again.

It is critical that we explore this process from a place of humility and empathy for ourselves and others. Attempts at mastery are a basic human way of coping with trauma. If we don't fully understand this, we may end up berating ourselves and blaming those who are victims of suffering. If we are open—and free of judgment—in considering how this dynamic may operate for us and for others, we gain precious insight. Even if we decide that trauma mastery isn't an issue for us, it's important to be compassionate when we work with colleagues for whom this may be a factor.

Trauma mastery emerges in our lives in three primary places: our activities, our relationships, and our choice of work. Let's start with activities. We may find trauma mastery if we consider where we are most determined to spend our time. For example, someone on a backpacking trip may contract hypothermia and damage his or her fingers or toes. That person may continue to go back to the same area year after year, hoping that this next time, nothing unfortunate will happen. We see trauma mastery behaviors frequently after natural disasters. Nine months after Hurricane Katrina, I discussed this concept in a workshop in New Orleans. One participant said, "Well, that's really stupid." After taking some time to gather her thoughts, her colleague Dina Benton spoke up. She said, "You know, if we really think about it, it's exactly what the majority of us are trying to do in New Orleans right now." She felt that simply by remaining in New Orleans, she and her colleagues were trying, in part, to regain control over circumstances that had stripped them and so many others of any familiar life or sense of self.

We can also look for trauma mastery in relationships. As one colleague of mine said, "It got to the point where I didn't have friends anymore, I had a caseload." You may have heard others in your life (or perhaps yourself) say, "I married my brother" or "I feel like I'm dating my mother." According to Linda Mooney, a medicine woman,

Native American spirituality regards this phenomenon as no accident. Instead of feeling confused and victimized by the challenging people who appear in our lives, her tradition teaches, we need to claim our role in inviting these people in. Mooney says we call into our lives the teachers we most need to learn from, and these teachers will reappear in person after person until we finally absorb the necessary lessons. This philosophy goes so far as to say we choose the families we are born into. Whether or not this is a belief you can adhere to, it can be invaluable to reassess the problematic people in our lives as teachers instead of tormentors. We can gain great wisdom if we acknowledge that we play a powerful part in our relationships. We can ask ourselves, "Have I been here before?" And if so, "What do I have left to learn?"

 Although firsthand experience with trauma leads to personal suffering, it can be sublimated into social or artistic action and thus can serve as a powerful agent for social change.

Bessel A. van der Kolk, clinician, researcher,
and teacher, Boston, Massachusetts

Finally, we often see trauma mastery in our choice of work and careers. This dynamic is one of the reasons why people stay in "helping professions," for example, even when they foresee a career of low-paying, difficult, and poorly resourced work. Some people feel driven to work in a field that is connected to an earlier trauma in their life; consciously or not, they intend to master the haunting echoes from a previous time. It may be the mother whose postpartum depression has lifted and who now leads support groups for new parents, the drought survivor who now champions international aid for regional water-well projects, or the law enforcement officer whose father was killed in the line of police duty. Someone reviewing incoming master of social work applications once told me that every single personal essay she had read to date cited a traumatic history as a primary factor in the applicant's decision to attend social work school.

Indeed, there are many leaders whose choice of their life's work was informed by trauma mastery. Rubin "Hurricane" Carter is an example. A professional boxer who was falsely convicted of murder and served two decades in prison, Carter is now a prominent advocate for those who are wrongly imprisoned. His hard-won wisdom and consciousness about what motivates him have helped him to make the world a better place. My own father's journey is also one of such reconciliation.

My parents were divorced at the time when my mother died of cancer, but they had previously been married for 20 years. My brother was 16 and I was 13. My father was self-employed, with a fulfilling career in public relations. Decades after my mother died, a PR assignment brought him in contact with a hospital program that was intended to help the children of people with cancer. Not long after his first meeting there, my father closed his public relations practice. He created a foundation dedicated to supporting children whose parents have cancer. He has worked on this issue nationally and internationally, and he has even compiled a book on the subject. Every day he brings a fierce passion and stunning commitment to his work. This commitment may best be understood by reading the dedication page in his book: "With love to my two great (grown) kids, Craig and Laura. I wish I had done more."

Some who are contending with trauma mastery as a dynamic in their work may find it difficult to separate what is now from what was then. Whether it is the refugee from Darfur, Sudan, who finds herself working for refugee rights or the child-abuse survivor who becomes a prosecuting attorney, people who have chosen a life's work based on trauma mastery will know in their bones that the stakes in what they do are exponentially high. Their expectations for themselves and others may be untenable and destructive. Continuing to explore all the ways trauma mastery may unfold in our lives personally and professionally is the first step toward awareness. Compassion for ourselves is critical. By developing a mindful and deliberate practice to heal from trauma, we take a proactive step. Around the world, we have countless role models—people who have been effective in repairing the world while still in the process of repairing their own hearts.

Sometimes the trauma we're hoping to master is so outside our reach that we work to heal ourselves by reconciling our pain in a distinct, yet related, effort. A colleague of mine was doing research on nonhuman primates and other large mammals deep in the rain forests of West Africa when a civil war broke out and disrupted his work. When he returned, he was unable to continue his work with animals, but he found another way to promote healing. "I don't know how to reconcile the past, but I suspect my reconciliation strategy is to merely move forward in seeking to do good works. Last summer I led a team of three ob-gyn surgeons to conduct several dozen obstetric fistula repairs at a rural hospital. No doubt, some of these were gynecological trauma due to the extreme forms of sexual violence inflicted during the war. For certain, the lives of several dozen women—total strangers to me—were transformed. This is what I mean by moving forward. I have come to believe that to get to the future, your path must pass through your nightmares. My time in West Africa taught me that lesson."

TRY THIS

1. Consider to what degree trauma mastery may be a factor in your work. As you ask yourself why you're doing this work, see if there are any historical wounds that motivate you.
2. If you think that trauma mastery is one reason you are drawn to your work, assess how else you are attending to this original trauma in other areas of your life. Are there additional ways to support your healing, thereby decreasing your potential dependence on your work in this regard?
3. Consider the people you know, either personally or through the

media, who have thoughtfully attended to trauma mastery as it applies to their work.

PROFILE ZAID HASSAN

LONDON, ENGLAND
CURRENTLY: Facilitator, writer, founder of Reos Partners, author of a book in progress on active responses to the destruction of cultures.
FORMERLY: Worked with Generon Consulting on long-term projects involving sustainable food supply chains in North America and Europe, child malnutrition in India, and aboriginal relations in Canada.

I think the place to start is with context, which for me is in my family more than anything else. Coming from a family where we've been refugees forever, I've grown up with this sentence in my head that no problem is really a problem. Ever since we've been kids, being upset about a problem or despairing or being depressed has just been a no-no. We were raised with an attitude that no problem is so big that it should be overwhelming, and for the longest time that was never really called into question. I think the last five or six years of work have made me really look at this.

My ancestors' and parents' history is part of my personal history, and every day I realize how much it's shaped the work I do. That might seem obvious, but it hasn't been obvious to me. Both sets of my grandparents lived in Calcutta and moved to East Pakistan in 1947 when Partition happened. That was the largest mass movement in history. It was a traumatic event, and our family lost everything in that move. And then in 1971 there was civil war between East and West Pakistan, and then my family was on the Bangladesh side and they had to flee to Karachi and again had to lose everything in the process. And then my family lived in the Middle East in the 1990s, and we basically had to flee from there in 1992 because my father had a disagreement with one of the local rulers. It has become a strange pattern, and we've carried a mindset or a set of beliefs that has come with those experiences. I haven't fully been able to explore what it all means or how it has affected me, but I know that it's there. I can see it through the mist, but I haven't cleared the mist away.

Working with Generon [a consulting firm that addresses intractable social issues around the globe, where Hassan worked at the time of our interview] has exposed me to situations that are very complex and stuck at one level and increasingly traumatic, so the work I'm getting increasingly involved with is around primary trauma. How secondary trauma and trauma stewardship come up is that we work with organizations where people have this suck-it-up attitude. So as an organization we in turn work incredibly long hours and have an incredibly demanding lifestyle of being on trains and planes all the time, and while we'd have the conversation about what is life balance, it never really resolved itself. For me the clarity came during a project in India, where I was working on malnutrition. In India as a team we re-created the sort of internal culture that Generon had. It was the hypermasculine work ethic of you never complain, you work 10 times as hard as you have to, and you never stop to pay attention to that culture and what it's doing to you. We re-created that in the culture of that project, and everyone became exhausted and wiped out all the time. The more tired people were, the less capable they were of dealing with complex issues in any way. The last day of this one series of three weeks was the single worst day I've ever had, workwise. It broke down in the group and it broke down amongst us and it was just awful.

I was debriefing that experience with one of my colleagues, and I was telling her about how we take people on nature solos where they go out into the woods alone. I told her how one of the guys had been gone for an hour in his tent and then couldn't be there alone, and afterwards we found out he'd had a really difficult childhood and teen years and a very traumatic past that he'd never dealt with. She asked, "What provisions have you made for folks when trauma surfaces at a psychosocial and at a personal level?" I realized we were just really lucky that nothing bad happened with this man. Her response was, "You can't have someone commit suicide on your project," and that really shook me up. I realized that we were unprepared and how much that was a reflection on our culture. I reflected a lot on India and how different it could have been if we'd paid attention to health for all of us. So for the last year I've been working on consciously building in processes for health and wellness.

At Generon, we knew what health and wellness processes were for, but only intellectually. In India, our thinking totally shifted from "These are dispensable practices" to "These are indispensable practices." If we want people working with empathy and care and to do this well, we have to build in practices around health and trauma. One thing that is becoming more and more important in our group work is the idea of embodiment—how do we embody in the space and in ourselves what we are doing? The problematic paradigms we work with manifest themselves in the physical all the time. You can work with them on the linguistic level—by talking about them—or you can work with them on the physical level. I'm interested in how we can shift these nonverbal paradigms that are the cause of systemic problems. If you have a certain policy that doesn't work or if you have a bunch of buildings that don't have windows, they are literal manifestations of what people believe are important and not important.

Another way is you actually shift the physical and see what impact that has. This is the idea of embodiment on the physical level: How do we carry ourselves, and how do our beliefs about health manifest in the room? It's a pretty uncomfortable thing for people to look at. In my experience, people are happy to look at anything that is outside the room. It's easy to look at problems in other communities, other practices. But to shift and look at ourselves—to look at how we are contributing to this in the moment—that takes a lot of courage and a lot of will. We typically think of systemic change as something that is happening far away from us. But things don't happen out there, they happen in the room. We just don't see them.

One experience I had came when we were doing a skit around people's lives in a community as part of a course. One of our colleagues teaches bodywork and dance, and she sprang up and said, "Let's look at what is really happening here." There was a guy standing up lecturing a group of people who were representing the community. She pointed out all the dynamics just in the placement of people's bodies. That was just a real insight into how power manifests in the room as a result of how we use our bodies, and how changing this can actually shift the power dynamics. One of the things we're tying into is that these power dynamics give rise to symptoms. "The system is perfectly designed to produce the results it does"—I keep hearing that quote. The frustrating part for me is that when you have a system that is producing a lot of trauma, people focus on that trauma, and there's very little attention focused on the source. What is this system that is churning out so many people who are suffering? I know there are not infinite resources, but if we could put even 10 percent of our resources into what is generating trauma, then we could make a difference. Otherwise, I think we're all going to just get overwhelmed.

I'm learning that it is incredibly hard to manifest all this in your own life. There is a huge burden of responsibility on the individual to shift things, and of course that's true—the individual is the first place it starts. Still, it's very, very hard to take responsibility for my own health when the systems and the culture around me are designed to provide minimal support for health. A terrific example is just trying to find healthy food while traveling. I've found it really interesting to try to shift my work patterns. For example, I have to travel a lot, and there's this expectation that I'm going to turn up even if I have to fly across the Atlantic for just one day. I started saying, "I'm not going to come." The reaction I initially got from colleagues was anger, and I really had to hold a line on that. They'd say, "It's important that you're there, this is urgent." And I'd have to say, "It's important for you, and I've got other priorities, unfortunately." It's hard to reprioritize your health in a context where people think that suicide in a community elsewhere is a bigger problem.

Understandably, people in the center of trauma feel there is nothing more urgent, and in one sense there isn't. But every conversation is about saving the world, and every conversation is about life and death. I just started saying no, you can't approach it that way. I had to realize that the world didn't end because I wasn't there. I think it's important to take a step back and ask, "Is it really necessary to be there?" It feels really great to have someone say, "We want you to fly across the Atlantic and be here," and we all want someone to say that to us, but it's also an illusion.

We need structures around us that will support us. Instead of working for an organization that can't provide that structure, I'm starting up my own organization. I'm trying to build in a healthy structure instead of grafting it on later. I'm a really strong believer that the pattern is set at the beginning, and you live in a pattern.

Last year for me got really, really full, and as a result I didn't have time to just do nothing. One of the things I did in response to that crazy year was I spent a week at home alone. That was hard and it was really, really, really good. It was great just being able to be with myself, to be comfortable with myself, and to allow whatever I wanted from within me to emerge. The first couple of days are hard; we have so much around us to distract us and there's this attitude we have toward inactivity. It's a huge privilege to be able to cultivate being with yourself, and it felt really grounding. So that's one of the things I'd like to do more regularly. I've been trying to take three days here and a week there, and I just wake up and see what happens. That generally works well. It's not a formal practice, but just having space makes a difference. To me, anyway.

Family is also a big part of it for me—being close to family and being in family. Family provides me with a context for a lot of learning and in some ways for building patience. The more we can build patience internally, the more we can build patience for complexity outside. It has been an interesting choice to live at home and deal with my family on a day-to-day basis. I'd noticed that the more my work affected me, the harder it was to be home. I'd turn up for a week after a trip for work, and my parents would say, "You're not here. Where are you?" I'd say, "I'm right here," and they'd say, "No, you're not. You're not really here." Ironically, my mom, who doesn't have any training in counseling and trauma, just sees through this really clearly. She's been calling this out for a long time. I think it'd be amusing for her that I have had to go through all these experiences and have all these professionals telling me what she's been telling me for a long time.

It's indispensable, following these practices of caring for myself. Even if they're difficult, they're indispensable. I just can't do the work I'm being called to do if I don't. And if I really believe what I've been saying about being present in the room, then I have to be present in the room. It's so easy to rush around and miss half the data. What you need to know is right there in front of you. If you're exhausted and uncoordinated and rushing around, you're just going to miss it. It's just human biology—you're just going to miss it.

My understanding of the work I'm doing has changed quite dramatically. You have social situations that have not improved for 50 or 500 years, and you need to figure out how to do something different. How do you support groups to choose a different pattern from the one they're in? I used to think this was about teaching new skills—creation, innovation, etc. I realize now that the work is about creating or opening a space and keeping it empty. What skills does it take to hold a space open so that the wisdom that is already there can come out? How can you be silent and sit with yourself and be compassionate and patient? A lot of what fills space is concern and fear and anxiety, and suspending those habitual reactions takes a lot of work. Slowing down, knowing your own patterns, and knowing what triggers you are a big part of that. On both a personal and an institutional level, people are petrified of empty space. It's like, fill the space, fill the space. There's a quote from Jung. Someone asked him, "Do you think we'll make it?" His answer was always the same: "We will if we do our inner work."

Is This Working for Me?

> My family would tell you that I'm resistant.... I know all of this, but I don't know that I want to change.
> Outreach worker helping victims of human trafficking

Once we are fluent in the language of why we are doing what we are doing, we can take the next step: asking ourselves, "Is this working for me?" As the answers to that question emerge, we can strategize about which elements to address, when, and how. (Figure 8.2)

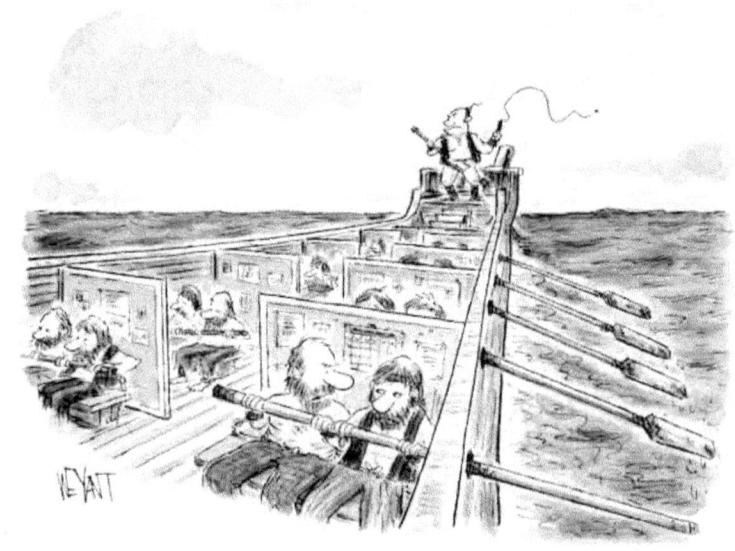

Figure 8.2: "I don't mind the whip. It's the cubicles I find demoralizing."

James Mooney led Native American Ceremonies for individuals struggling with a broad range of life's challenges. People flew in from around the country to work with him and his wife. The Ceremonies lasted all day and sometimes all night. People would sit across from Mooney and describe their lives and specific situations. He would tend to his burning sage and cedar and listen. Then he'd look up at them and ask, "Does that work for you?" He posed the question casually, but like

Jorge Alvarado he was actually cutting through all the surface layers of a person's situation: the helplessness we feel under the weight of not-rightness in our lives, the dishonesty we perpetuate within ourselves to resist the risk of change, the ways we contort our true selves to conform to perceived, often distorted ideals. Really he was asking, "Who are you? Please get honest and connect with your heart."

For Mooney, the more simply you spoke, the more honest you were. When I first started working with him, I answered his question with a long, convoluted, hyperintellectual response. He looked back calmly at me and said, "Sweetheart, I have a third-grade education. I can't understand anything you're saying." And so I'd try again, and again, and again. And it was only when I was able to muster the courage to be totally honest with myself and with him that my answer became intelligible, because it was from my heart and not from my head. What I was saying finally made sense.

Somewhere along the way, many of us doing work we believe to be of great value to society find that it's really not working for us. It can be very hard to admit this. At one time in our life, certain actions and choices may help us to survive or serve our well-being. Then, as we evolve as people, we often come to realize that these behaviors—which we thought were essential to us—are no longer in our best interest. It can be incredibly difficult to change, because these patterns may be a part of our identity, and we're likely to have relied on them extensively. Still, as a qigong healer once told me, "This is no longer helping you. This is only harming you now. Are you ready to put this down?"

I have found that it is critical, when asking yourself this question, to be free of self-judgment and to try to be honest in your assessment. Remember that the effects of work on our lives may show up in very small or extremely large forms. As you try to open yourself to the truth, frame the question in various ways. "Does it work for me? How does it work for me? Why does it work for me?" And once you've answered these questions, more will follow: "Am I doing my work with integrity, given all this? Are my reasons for doing this ethical?"

I have heard many people say that they embrace their work in part because it reinforces a worldview they have clung to over time. Upon exploring her trauma exposure response, an advocate for victims of human trafficking remarked, "Actually, I think this work has just made what was already there in my personality much more extreme." Similarly, a public interest attorney said, "I've never been a glass-is-half-full kind of a guy, and this work has just reinforced my cynicism." The echo effect is compelling, but it often reinforces pain and negativity. It can be a hard cycle to break.

On the other hand, work provides many people with a means to fix what they see as broken in the world. It can be a relief to find likeminded colleagues who will work toward a shared goal, especially when that goal involves rectifying injustice. Many of us are raised in communities where the social norms encourage us to minimize conflict, disguise suffering, and ignore disparity.

While the rubble of the World Trade Center still smoldered, then-president George Bush implored us to go shopping as a testimony to our nation's resolve. Not to grieve, not to be kind to each other, not to reflect deeply and humbly on the series of wounds and tragedies that preceded the hijackers' confoundingly violent and hopeless attacks, not to pitch in and make a difference in our own communities, but to shop. While this comment has often been remarked upon, it remains a shining example of how distracted and numbed-out our culture and governance can become. It also indicates how alienating it can be to work for social and environmental justice. For many people, it can be crazy-making and lonely to see that there are tangible causes of suffering, but at the same time to be surrounded by people who are committed to obliterating any such awareness from their—and our—consciousness.

This is in part what was so mind-blowing about the early years of feminism in the United States. At last, all the unnamed things that women had experienced as a result of centuries of sexism were given names, explained, and made visible. For a time, no one needed to feel alone or crazy anymore. It is similar to how former U.S. vice president Al Gore may feel in the present day as he champions the cause of global-warming awareness. He explains in his film, *An Inconvenient Truth,* "You know, there are a lot of people who go straight from denial to despair without pausing on the intermediate step of actually doing something about the problem." The film shows how, in the midst of a global climate crisis, his path is truly working for him and bringing him a great deal of hope.

Striving to make the world a better place, then, works for some people because they can find larger structures and movements that allow them to enjoy life while also tending to what needs tending. It is similar to the inspiration and sustenance that you may feel when someone like Noam Chomsky or Ray Suarez or Vandana Shiva or Barack Obama gives voice to something you care deeply about. It can help balance other responses to your work, which may be along the lines of, "Oh, that is so depressing! How do you do that kind of thing?"

It takes courage to admit that our work may no longer be working for us. A friend and colleague of mine, Zaid Hassan, is often invited to help improve social situations that are entrenched and detrimental. He attends to them, sometimes for years, until some transformation can take place. He has served a broad array of those in need, from orphans in India to AIDS victims in South Africa to First Nations communities. He told me about his efforts in Canada, where he tried to address issues of suicide, substance abuse, and domestic violence. On his flight home to London, he finally took the time to catch up on the e-mail that had been accumulating for weeks: "And there I read in an e-mail that had been sent two weeks prior that a friend of mine's brother had killed himself back home. I sat there reading it and could not believe that my friend had reached out to me during this time of such pain and I had not been available to him, even as I was working for a solution to decrease suicide rates halfway around the world. I decided right then that I never wanted something like this to happen again, where I would be too consumed by my work to attend to a friend in need."

When we gain insight into the *why* of our work and we find specific parts that *do* work for us, it can feel like a tremendous gift. As John Brookins, now a prison reentry specialist and a men's ministry director, shared, "I'm right where I want to be. I wish I had been here earlier, but as a Black Panther I was too angry to undo racism. Now, with some more age and maturity, I can really be present with my work in the prisons. I think to myself: 'I can do this. We can do this. This is possible.' I'm right where I want to be."

Viktor Frankl, in his book *Man's Search for Meaning,* focuses on the task of finding a calling that serves us while we serve others. He says that understanding what one is meant to do is worth the hardship that often surrounds the seeking: "What man actually needs is not a tensionless state but the striving and struggling for a worthwhile goal, a freely chosen task.... If architects want to strengthen a decrepit arch, they increase the load that is laid upon it, thereby joining the parts more firmly together." So while the exploration of "Is this working for me?" may temporarily *increase* our load, in the long term we will be more stable as a result of addressing the question.

TRY THIS

1. Brainstorm five ways in which you think what you are doing is working for you.
2. Take three deep breaths and review your list. Assess to what degree those ways are or are not in your best interest or the best interest of those you serve.
3. Create a list of five ways in which you would ideally see your work benefiting you and those you serve. Compare the two lists.

CHAPTER NINE

EAST • Choosing Our Focus

As we move to the east, we call upon the new life and enlightenment of the fire element, which is revered in many cultures as the keeper of truth and originator of all energy. We ask ourselves where we're putting our focus, and we expand our range of possibilities by imagining a Plan B. We gain a new sense of freedom by understanding that we have the ability to shift our perspective. When we open ourselves to inspiration, we may also rediscover our passion. This is the perfect moment to be honest about what we are able to accomplish in our existing job and what our options might be.

Where Am I Putting My Focus?

> The real voyage of discovery consists not in seeking new landscapes but in having new eyes.
> Marcel Proust, French intellectual and novelist

Being conscious of where we are putting our focus can teach us that we have incredible freedom in how we choose to interact with our lives. I was reminded of this during recent travels in Mexico. I attempted to learn how to surf and now realize why, for the majority of surfers, it is a religion, a philosophy, a way of life. Awestruck, I suddenly understood surfing, or our ability to ride the waves, as a metaphor for life.

You're out in the wide-open ocean, hoping to catch a wave. You can be annoyed that the sets are so far apart and the waves are breaking from the wrong direction—or you can choose to notice that the sky is blue and the sun is out and you're with a whole group of strangers who are loving the waiting. Then the waves arrive, and you have no control over them. Wave after wave comes, in surfing as in life, and you don't get to decide what they look like or how they break or how far apart they are. What you do get to choose is which wave you try to catch, which wave you are going to focus on.

When you pick a wave, you try your best. Sometimes you ride it all the way in and it's sublime. Often you ride it for a time and you fall off, sometimes very hard. In that moment, as in life, you have a decision to make. Do you focus on the seconds that you stayed upright, rejoice that there will be another wave to catch, feel blessed that you are in a position to try for a wave at all? Or do you belittle yourself for not being strong enough, curse the wave, blame another surfer, or tell yourself that if the board handled differently, you would have had a different ride? It is always up to us where we place our focus. It is this choice that will determine, ultimately, what our ride is like. (Figure 9.1)

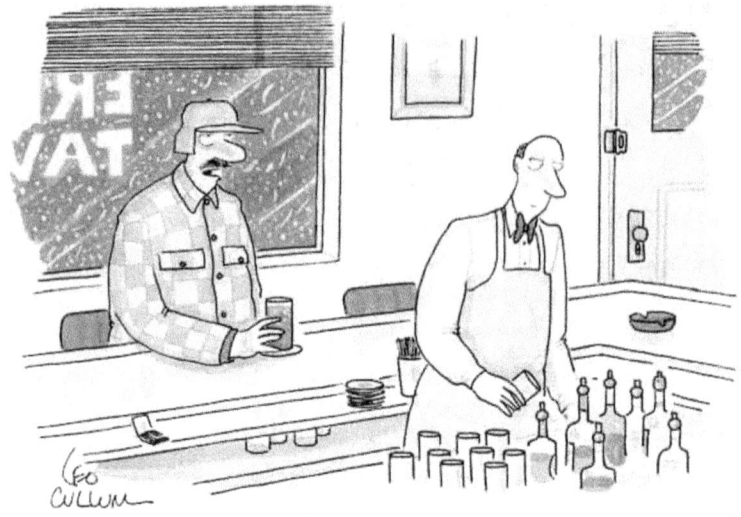

Figure 9.1: "May I have a tiny umbrella in this, Ernie? I'm on vacation."

This teaching is shared throughout the world. The Indian doctor and spiritual teacher Deepak Chopra describes life as a series of scenes revealing themselves; in every moment, we decide where to place our attention. Focusing on negative, painful, troubling events can become habitual. It takes discipline to raise our gaze; look away from our accustomed pain, anxiety, and worries; and truly see the world through different eyes.

Rubin "Hurricane" Carter once said to Lesra Martin, "It is very important to transcend the places that hold us....

When I started writing, I discovered that I was doing more than just telling a story.... Every time I sat down to write, I could rise above the walls of this prison. I could look out over the walls all across the state of New Jersey, and I could see Nelson Mandela in his cell writing his book. I could see Huey. I could see Dostoyevsky. I could see Victor Hugo, Emile Zola. It's magic..." No matter how uncontrollable and torturous our external world may be, we remain sovereign over what we focus on. We can change our lives by reframing our experiences.

> I focus on what I was able to do that day. I focus on what went well, what changed, what moved, and what I was able to do. And the rest, the rest I leave behind at the end of the day.

Pediatrician in a community health clinic

In the field, reframing may take different forms. Sometimes it means concentrating on what's in front of you, and sometimes it means stepping back. If one client dies, you may need to remember all the others who have lived.

If it is the world that seems overwhelming, it may be better to concentrate on individuals. Street Yoga is an organization in Portland, Oregon, that supports homeless youth and the providers who serve them by teaching yoga, meditation, and wellness classes. When it came time to write a new mission statement, they took great care not to strive for something that would leave them perpetually feeling like they weren't doing enough. Even amid the overwhelming reality that homeless youth face, they have found a way to focus on something that is, indeed, within reach. It reads, "Street Yoga is working to ensure that every person is at home in their own body, their own mind, and their own community, and that no one is ever homeless again."

Resourcing, as it's called in the field of somatic experiencing, is a concrete way to work with focus. If you feel either suddenly or chronically out of balance, you can regroup by remembering your "resources"—the moments, people, places, and experiences that engage your parasympathetic nervous system, which is primarily engaged during times of rest. You might call up an image or memory that brings you peaceful and joyful sensations, for example. You might also take note that there is no immediate crisis: At least for the moment, the earth is not shaking, court is adjourned, surgery is over, the grant application is done, and so on. If you allow yourself this break, your system will begin to calm and regulate itself. Your heart rate slows, your breathing gets deeper, and the adrenaline slowly subsides. As you notice this, remind yourself that you can come back to a place of homeostasis.

It can be as simple, yet helpful, as the technique that a skilled practitioner shared with me when I was describing my distress over a persistent cough. Instead of concentrating solely on the discomfort near the front of my chest, she said, "Let's bring your awareness to your back. How does the back of your chest feel? What about the other lung, how does that feel?" Through such mental efforts, we can achieve increased calm and balance. The more we practice coming into the present moment and focusing on our internal and external resources, the more skills we will have to care for ourselves when we experience either acute or chronic stress.

There is great power in understanding that we can change the way we interact with circumstances in our lives, simply by being intentional about where we put our focus. Daniel Siegel and Jack Kornfield, one a scientist and the other a Buddhist monk, are beginning to teach this as they combine the latest in brain physiology research with the oldest of mindfulness practices. They explain that the way you pay attention activates parts of your brain in very specific ways, and that this brain firing actually leads to structural changes in the brain itself. In other words, there is a real likelihood that with time and practice, a temporary, intentionally created mindful state will become a lasting mental trait. However small the ways in which we bring awareness to where we're putting our focus may seem, they can lead to large changes in our experience of life. William James, a pioneering American philosopher and psychologist who was trained as a medical doctor, said, "My experience is what I agree to attend to."

Several years ago, Seattle's Environmental Home Center burned to the ground. A wonderful resource for renewable, sustainable, and green building products was destroyed, at least for a time. The postcard that the company sent out after the fire, which appears below, illustrates an enlightened approach to the hardship. (Figure 9.2)

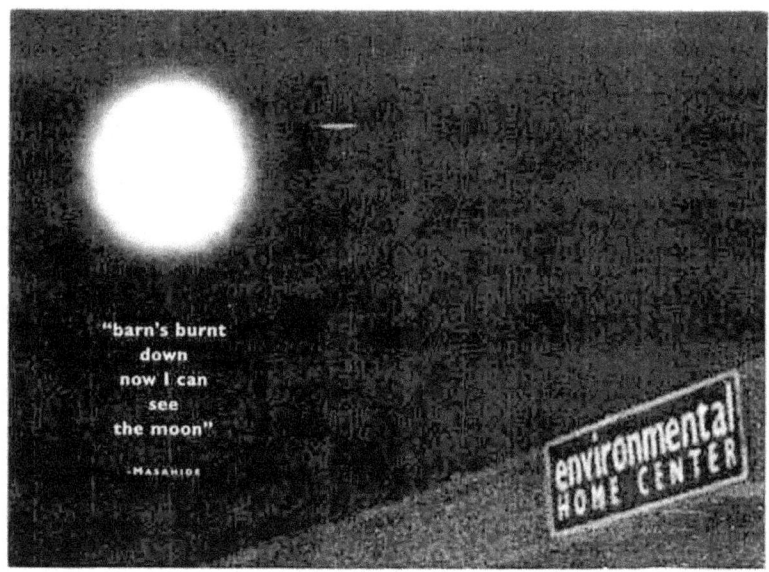

Figure 9.2

TRY THIS

1. Think of a challenging work situation. Write down three things that make it challenging. Write down three things that you appreciate about it. Look at your lists and ask yourself, "Where am I more likely to focus and why?"
2. For one day, commit to paying attention to the running commentary in your mind. Is your mind in the habit of seeing the glass as half-empty or half-full? Are you able to reframe things as half-full, or do you feel an investment in seeing things as half-empty?
3. Find a mirror, stand in front of it, and look at yourself. Notice the first three things that come to mind. Would you classify them as positive, loving, kind things? If not, try again.

PROFILE HELEN HOWELL
SEATTLE, WASHINGTON

CURRENTLY: Attorney/consultant

FORMERLY: National delegate and chair of Washington State Obama delegation, distinguished practitioner in residence at Seattle University's School of Law, legal counsel to U.S. Senator Patty Murray, special assistant and deputy staff secretary to President Bill Clinton, vice president for public policy at Planned Parenthood Federation of America, deputy chief of staff for Governor Gary Locke of Washington.

My sister and I have had conversations about why we're doing what we're doing; why we have this real-life fantasy that work is something that is supposed to be enjoyable and meaningful. I think it came from watching my father go off to work each day. As children, we thought he was going off to play, because he liked what he did so much. [Helen Howell's father, Lem Howell, is a longtime civil rights activist as well as a renowned personal injury attorney in Seattle.] I think that explains a lot about my unduly high expectations about what work is to provide in one's life. I have all these criteria that my work must meet. It must be stimulating and challenging, and it has to matter. I need to feel like I am making a difference, that I am contributing to making the world better.

I must enjoy it, though, because I keep doing it. I have had a series of very intense, time-limited jobs, the kind that consume one's whole life. While it was very, very exciting, I was miserable personally. Then you look up and seven years are gone. It takes a pretty profound toll on you when you're unhappy. I have tremendous capacity, and I got a tremendous amount of satisfaction from my work. I could have gone on working like that for years, but I had some kind of realization that this can't be it ... Work can't be it alone. There has to be more to life.

I used to think that you weren't working unless you were totally spent, unless you walked in the door and crashed on your couch. But then I went to work in the governor's office. There were people there who were completely devoted and dedicated, and they also had to catch their carpool shuttle at 4:30. I'd look around and think: It's not even lunchtime. Where's everyone going? Why am I and my one colleague the only ones here? What's our deal that we're still here? Once I had my daughter, I realized that maybe I could do other things in my life. Maybe I could be a parent. If you are going to be who you want to be as a parent, you clearly have to have some energy at the end of the day.

A turning point for me was a few months after my daughter was born, when she developed a respiratory virus. It was shortly after I returned to work. She was hospitalized for three days, and while I think I made one call to the chief of staff at the time, I didn't do anything else, workwise. There was no you should do this or that, or you need to do this and that—none of it. This far outweighed anything else, and everyone I worked with understood, and nobody put any pressure on me. But more significant for me was that I was totally present and right there, and for once I didn't have to assess what my priorities were. It just happened. I was totally present, and that was really amazing to me. I came to understand that I had a capacity I didn't know I had, which was to completely suspend my work life. And from there I came to understand that not everyone works at 110 percent capacity, and that maybe it's not normal to operate like that. I had been very unrealistic about that. It was a flash point for me to recognize that I'd been living life in a way that was super-intense.

I was raised like a lot of Black kids, where I internalized that you have to be twice as good to get half as far and that I have a responsibility to others. The belief that to whom much is given, much is expected. I also grew up in an immigrant family with a father whose life was a Horatio Alger story. And I watched my mom, a martyr who remains the most radical person I know in terms of her political beliefs, but who struggled to take care of herself personally. I grew up internalizing how my parents had been impacted by the British colonization of their homeland in Jamaica in the West Indies; they were preoccupied with what is and is not appropriate and what one should do. Plus for Dad, between the navy and the law, life was full of rules. And I grew up continually reminded of how blessed and lucky I was, given all the suffering in the world. I have internalized this stuff, this sense of what I should be doing to contribute to the world, to the point that it is who I am. Sometimes I get tired of feeling like I'm endlessly searching, and I wonder what my journey is about. In my heart, I believe it's about arriving at a place where I feel that I can realize my greatest potential, but that's quite a recipe, I suppose, and I don't know when it will be enough.

As an African-American woman, when I talk to people, I don't get any automatic credibility or assumptions of competence. And the things that I work on aren't valued greatly by society, so already I'm living in a world that doesn't respect what is important to me. There is a feeling of being ultimately undervalued, but I worry about moving into that area of feeling persecuted. And the work itself, in the advocacy world, it's tough. It's difficult to make the decisions you have to make knowing the large-scale impact they'll have on the lives of others. There is tremendous responsibility involved. And then there are the value dynamics and conflicts that surface. Even with coalition partners, we don't always or even often agree on what is best for our nation, the people of the state of Washington, women, low-income people, or people of color.

I have carried that weighty baggage with me. But you're not

going to complain. Intense in my family was when something was dire. A real problem when my dad was growing up was when you didn't know where your next meal was going to come from or when you lost your mother at the age of 10. Then when you work for the president of the United States, you see his schedule. He was booked from 7a.m. to 11p.m., and then he'd be reading a book or two on top of it. He was working even harder than we were, so it was all OK. It's such important work and we have only so much time. You're always carrying it. It's continual. Even when you're off and if you're watching the news, you're thinking about what the plan will be and what that means for tomorrow.

What Is My Plan B?

I was always dreaming. Dreaming, dreaming, always dreaming. Those weren't easy times, but I never stopped dreaming.

Rollie Dick, an American schoolteacher and principal for 40 years who retired to Mexico and opened a restaurant with local townspeople

When we realize the degree to which we can determine our focus, we may also open to the possibility that we have more options about how we structure our lives and work than we may have thought. To deepen this awareness, I often encourage people in my workshops to dream up a new vision for how they might conduct their lives. In other words, to create a Plan B.

Like most of the exercises I suggest in this book, developing a Plan B can be both powerful and unsettling—to you and the people around you. As I was completing a workshop on trauma stewardship for a gathering of heads of independent schools in the Pacific Northwest, one gentleman raised his hand and said, "I have to be honest. Part of me is sitting here thinking about how quickly can I get you to come train all my colleagues back home. And part of me is thinking that you are the last person in the world I want to set foot on the school campus. I can't afford to have everyone I work with leave. If they have too much opportunity to think about their options, they might decide to do something different."

Having a Plan B reminds us that what we do is an act of free will. Plan B could involve a career change, a new place to live, a fresh approach to our current work, or a different life altogether. It may be frightening to consider any departure from what we know. But even if we never go ahead with our Plan B, the mere act of considering alternatives may create an opening to broaden our conception of our life's work.

While it may be difficult to envision a Plan B, it is a practice worth trying. We can be so overwhelmed by logistics, minutiae, and the perceived constraints in our lives that we can see our work as a burden, an imposition, something being done to us. Through creating and re-creating a Plan B, we come to understand that it is we who make the fundamental choices about the work we do. While there is great responsibility that comes with this understanding, there is tremendous freedom as well. We always have options to change what we do, where we do it, or how we approach the work at hand. (Figure 9.3)

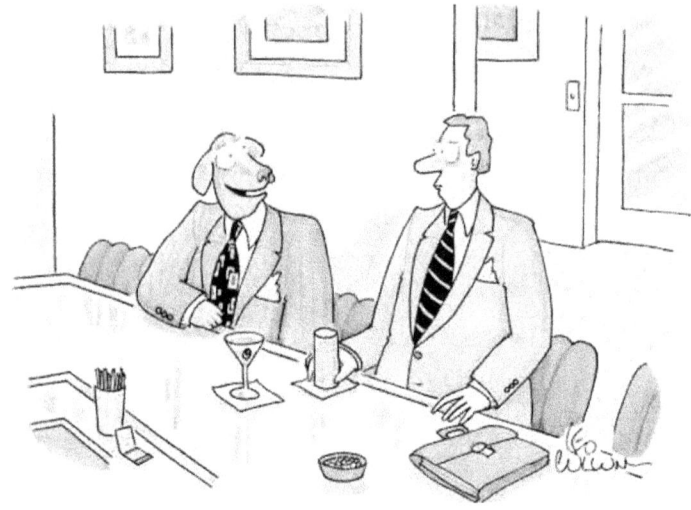

Figure 9.3: "Selective breeding has given me an aptitude for the law, but I still love fetching a dead duck out of freezing water."

This knowledge may serve us in profound ways. As Viktor Frankl writes, "Man can preserve a vestige of spiritual freedom, of independence of mind, even in such terrible conditions of psychic and physical stress. We who lived in concentration camps can remember the men who walked through the huts comforting others, giving away their last piece of bread. They may have been few in number, but they offer sufficient proof that everything can be taken from a man but one thing: the last of the human freedoms—to choose one's attitude in any given set of circumstances, to choose one's own way."

There are smaller psychic rewards for having a Plan B as well. When you share dreams with colleagues and loved ones, their attention may remind you that life is filled with possibilities. A coworker may bring in an article on gardening for you, or a friend may pass on a report about expatriates living in South America. These are gifts that remind you that your core self is not what you do for work. Rumi, the 13th-century Persian jurist, theologian, and poet, wrote, "Let yourself be silently drawn by the stronger pull of what you really love."

In the late 1980s, Mike Ternasky helped found H Street skateboards. While he built a successful company with several friends as business partners, they had a saying around the office: "If this thing doesn't work out, we're gonna do Plan B." When Ternasky grew restless at H Street, he did indeed get rolling with Plan B, which created a team of top riders and "took the skateboard world by storm," as the company's Web site put it.

While I often encourage people to think about a Plan B far from their current field of work, I appreciate the degree to which a Plan B, even as it applies to our current work, can help us. A Plan B does not need to be a completely different lifestyle; it can be as subtle as a change in our attitude and the way we approach our existing commitments. (Figure 9.4)

Figure 9.4

It may be helpful to remind ourselves that the change we want in the world is not tied to any given profession. Moreover, we as individuals cannot be either completely limited or fully actualized in any one job. Each job is only one of millions of tools that can be used to achieve the larger goal. If I am fixing something, and for a while I need to use a hammer, no one will say I am failing if later I pick up a screwdriver. When we undertake a repair, we expect to need a whole box of tools. As we work, however, many of us come to think of our jobs as ends in themselves, and not merely as means to institute the change we seek. We become very attached to doing that exact work in that exact place. We worry that if we stop doing that job (using that tool), we will be forced to give up on the project of repair altogether.

It is counterproductive to think about various fields in terms of hierarchy or competition. It is a legacy of oppression that tells us we are "selling out" if we don't work for a nonprofit or stay on the front lines doing extreme work. We don't need to collude with the impoverished imagination that would have us believe there are only certain ways to contribute to the betterment of the world.

As Connie Burk has said, "I have discovered that at my core self there is a will to compassion. I've been amazingly fortunate to have a job where the connection between my paid work and this will is very explicit. But when I stop doing my current work, I will not be exempt from the task of right action. No matter what I do in the future, I will need to maintain that connection between what I do each day and my core will." As the work of the 19th-century American philosopher and abolitionist Frederick Douglass teaches us, compassion can be more than just a reaction to others' suffering. It can be proactive, something that you do as a matter of conscious choice.

Getting to know what our deepest will is in life can help us hugely in developing a Plan B and C and D. (Figure 9.5)

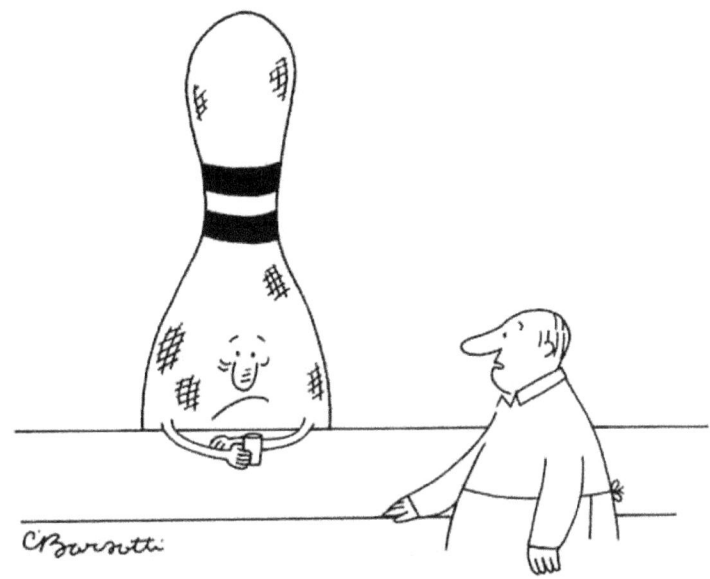

Figure 9.5 "Have you ever considered another line of work?"

TRY THIS

1. Ask yourself, "If I weren't doing this work, what would I love to do?"
2. Generate a list of five things you can do over the next five weeks to help you get closer to realizing your Plan B.
3. Tell three loved ones about your Plan B and ask them to encourage you in that direction at least once a month.

CHAPTER TEN

SOUTH • Building Compassion and Community

To the south we call upon the peace and renewal that come from the earth element. By developing a microculture of supportive friends and family, we create an environment that sustains us, just as the earth does. By being compassionate to ourselves and others, we ground ourselves. This is where we come out of isolation, tap into the core energies of Mother Nature, and tend to both our individual and collective health and wellness.

Creating a Microculture

Nearly every Sunday I get together with my family and we have soul food. My aunt is retired and she starts cooking early in the morning. Sometimes you can find four generations gathered together to share stories of our past and present. Over a period of time I started to notice that my workweek just seemed to flow better because I was starting Monday happy and relaxed.

>Charlann Hartfield, antipoverty advocate, Seattle, Washington

Whether you call it your sangha (the Sanskrit word for community or assembly), your consultation group, your women's group, your bar mates, or your circle of friends, it is critical to create a *microculture* of support around you. A microculture is simply a community, but I like the term because it reminds us that our chosen group may nurture us by emphasizing a different set of values than the culture at large.

In *The Dance of Change,* Peter Senge talks about "conscious oversight," an idea he borrowed from the Quakers: "In any Quaker community there is an oversight committee who is charged with enhancing the total health and sustainability of the community. Early writings state, 'desirable as it is that some would be specifically entrusted with these oversight duties, an earnest concern has prevailed that all may take their right share in the privilege of watching out for one another's good.'" Senge describes conscious oversight as being, in part, about slowing down "enough to reflect on the system and situation from a variety of perspectives and with a variety of ways of thinking. Also ... to bring an ongoing deliberation into everyone's frame of reference and to support them to take the long view in the midst of day to day." (Figure 10.1)

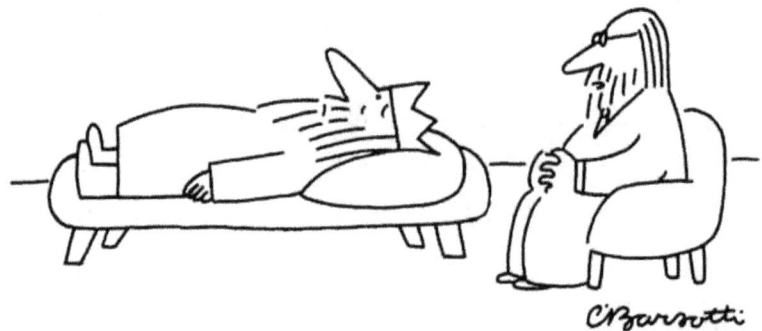

Figure 10.1: "Enemies, yes, but doesn't your moat also keep out love?"

Our microculture should support us in two ways: by showering us with encouragement and by holding us accountable. Its members must be people we can debrief with, laugh with, brainstorm with, consult with, cry with, and become better people with. Isolation is an underpinning of oppression, and by consciously staying connected with others, we are taking an important step toward trauma stewardship. In shamanic traditions throughout the world, communities recognize the critical need for social cohesion in tending to suffering and healing pain and trauma. Often rituals involve the entire community, and the integrating of individuals or a group back into themselves and the larger social fabric takes the form of song, dance, and ultimately celebration.

An important role of the community we create around us is to refuse to collude with our harmful internal patterns. There is a First Nations tribe on the coast of British Columbia, Canada, and like many Native communities, it will come together when someone asks to have a Circle. Anyone in the community can request a Circle, either to celebrate something or to ask for help. In this particular community, there has been an understanding: If someone in the community asks for a Circle, you show up. But it doesn't stop there. There is an agreement that if you realize as you listen that you've been called to this Circle more than once before—in other words, that the same person is asking for help on the same matter for the third time—then you will get up and move 20 feet over. The entire Circle will rise and follow you. The person who'd hoped to revisit the struggle yet again will have to decide if he/she wants to sit alone or if he/she is willing to move on and join the new Circle. "Move the Circle" is now a common expression among my family and friends. We say it whenever it seems that one of us has been ruminating on something long enough.

In the book *Traumatic Stress,* Marten W. deVries states: "Culture cannot prevent calamity, nor can it blunt the immediate physical power of violence and the emotional shock of betrayal. It can only help with building up resilience before such events, or with providing validation, restitution, and rehabilitation afterward. Cultural processes such as social support and self-help groups are powerful forces for restitution particularly when combined with formal cultural acceptance of the traumatic experience."

> In my family, we have a rule that anyone can call for a family hug at any time. It doesn't matter what you're caught up in—if you hear someone say 'family hug,' you stop everything you're doing and you go join in. We just take that moment to hold each other and be together, and then we all go back to doing what we were doing.
>
> First Nations health care worker

In one model project, microcultures are used to foster the reconciliation of trauma. Rebuild, a program of the Inova Regional Trauma Center in Virginia, supports individuals, families, and communities along the entire journey from traumatic incident to trauma stewardship. Recovering patients help each other deal with the long-term consequences of their injuries through support groups, self-management classes, and mentoring of new patients. In addition, these patients provide trainings to first responders and other health care professionals, including doctors, nurses, social workers, firefighters, and rehabilitation specialists. During these presentations, Rebuild members describe their experiences with the rescue, hospitalization, and rehabilitation processes, providing valuable insight into the profound journey shared by all trauma patients.

Recovering trauma patients can attend forums where they sit together and thank the paramedics, nurses, doctors, and therapists for their important role in the healing process. They also provide feedback about their experiences, which allows for closure and growth for both patient and caregiver. Reconnecting with patients has a profound effect on the caregivers; in a survey, they reported gaining valuable insights and feeling a renewed commitment to their chosen professions. A frequent comment was, "This is why I became a paramedic (firefighter, nurse, therapist, and so on): to truly make a difference in people's lives."

I, for one, believe that if you give people a thorough

understanding of what confronts them and the basic causes that produce it, they'll create their own program, and when the people create a program, you get action.
Malcolm X, American Black nationalist leader and founder of the Organization of Afro-American Unity

TRY THIS

1. Ask yourself what your ancestors and those who raised you have done, throughout time, to heal themselves and others. When they experienced trauma, how did they go on?
2. Identify the members of your microculture. To what degree do they nurture hopefulness, accountability, and integrity? Think about whether you could use stronger role models in any of these areas.
3. Take some time to examine how your outside surroundings connect with your internal state. Are there

shifts you can make in your external reality to achieve a more peaceful and productive internal reality? What is your neighborhood like, how is your home taken care of, what food do you eat, and what role do you choose in creating wellness both locally and globally?

PROFILE ANNA BRADFORD

VIENNA, VIRGINIA
CURRENTLY: Doctoral student, Johns Hopkins School of Public Health.
FORMERLY: Rebuild coordinator, Inova Regional Trauma Center.

The initial trauma in my life was when my friend Hilary died when I was a teenager. I think the actual evening when all of this happened was as shocking and horrible and difficult to understand as any other trauma, and I think it was managed as any other trauma in anyone's life is managed. From that experience, I feel like I have an understanding of what it is like to go through something that horrible and scary and gross and frightening and overwhelming. What is different about my experience, however, is that when Hilary's family did regroup, we were able to integrate this tragedy into who we were as a larger community. I believe today that I can have some impact in people's lives because of what my experience was personally in relation to this tragedy.

The way the Plancks decided how they wanted the funeral to be was incredibly significant in how we were able to integrate what had happened. They decided they wanted to bury their daughter on our farm, which they did in part because they wanted the process to be one that the community could be engaged in, so that everyone who'd been a part of her life could be a part of grieving her death together. She was brought home from the hospital, and while there was nothing different from how they did burials back in the day, it was very organic feeling. We were able to be very present with her and had an ability to hang out with her and touch and see her or not as we chose, but the way we handled the whole burial and processing was nicely paced, drawn out, over the course of a day or so. People decided together how to make the box for her, and they found the place to dig the hole. It actually takes a long time to dig a hole that big when you're doing it with a shovel. We decided together which of the things we'd made for her would go in the coffin. We were all working together. The whole funeral was all very organic: you show up and then we figure out what to do. Nothing was preordained. We'd take the time we needed to find some nails, and then we had to figure out how to carry this big box over to the hole we'd dug, and after we had buried her we knew that we now would have some time to hang out and talk about her and be together and have some food together. It felt very genuine instead of something we felt like we should be doing.

Then, in terms of us having time to integrate the burial and talk about it and have it not be such a bizarre thing, I'm not sure how well we did it in those months after the funeral. Her family had previously made plans to move away to another farm, and I had been scheduled to change schools. So they ended up moving, and when I changed schools I made a cognitive decision to not tell anyone what had just happened to me. When you don't talk about the biggest thing that is going on in your entire life, you figure out another person to be, and then eventually you become that other person. And on some level I realize now that I took this opportunity to adopt some of the same characteristics that Hilary had, that I definitely did not have. She had a very cheerful, intelligent, outgoing, positive personality, and that was what I took on as my personality. It took me over 10 years to look back on that time and realize that this transformation in me had happened.

Another thing that was distinct about what we did as a community was we got together around 15 years after her death. Her younger sister was going through a lot of challenges not uncommonly associated with someone who has experienced a great loss. Some of the process that had been so helpful to us 15 years prior was not particularly age-appropriate for her at the time, so she had inadvertently been excluded on some level. Her parents planned a gathering that was essentially a debriefing, which managed to include almost every person who had been present at the scene of the accident. It took a long time to schedule, because people were scattered around the country and around the world, but her parents just made it happen. What we did followed almost to the letter what you'd do in a critical incident stress debriefing, but I didn't realize that for another 10 years. The first person talked about what actually happened; we went through the specific details chronologically. Everyone shared what they remembered about the facts of the case. That probably took more than an hour. After that, we pieced together the pieces—and really, this was something, because it never occurred to me that everyone else was having their exact experience of dealing with her death as well for all those years. Then we were able to go through how it affected us at the time and have everyone express how that particular experience had influenced them for the rest of their life.

It was really a unique thing to have two families willing to do this thing together, and these two families were so good at it. It was so helpful to be able to name things. I was able to name how I felt like she continued to live in me. I remember having some sense of guilt about various things that I'd been carrying around all those years, and then everyone was totally accepting of it, and they also had their own things that they felt guilty about. Everyone was so honest that those elements then moved away. It was a great relief to have the blessing of her family in relation to all of our feelings, and to have them be so overjoyed to know that I felt like I was a continuing expression of who she was in many ways. It meant so much to all of us to have everyone's blessing and to have no judgment about how we handled our recovery. It probably lasted more than four hours, and it was considerably more invigorating than exhausting. We literally had to drag ourselves away. I mean, how do you leave something like that? We had to acknowledge that we had to go back to living our lives, and that's a hard thing to do.

After that, I knew that this had to be a part of what I do. I never had any idea that I'd go back to school. I eventually went to school to be a social worker. When I heard that social workers were placed in trauma settings, I remember thinking, "The only thing that has to happen in my life is that I have to be in the ER." I remember sitting there, and it's funny to me how incredibly obvious it was that there was nowhere else for me to be. I knew it didn't matter if I got paid or if they were able to give me any hours to work, I was like, "I have to be there." It was the only thing that was an option for me. I didn't realize why until four or five years later, when I was working there full time and I was talking with a student of mine, and I was telling her that I didn't really know how I'd ended up in trauma. Somehow we started talking about Hilary's death, and this student helped me connect my previous experiences with this work I was doing in my current program, which I was developing at the time. It had been very much unstated and unobserved. I never connected it. When my student first started making the connections for me, I was like, "Well, this is a bit of a stretch," but then another 10 years after that, I'm like, "Yeah, right!" and finally the puzzle pieces fell more into place.

In a way, the whole grieving experience we went through probably felt so natural because people have been doing this since trauma has been happening. There just wasn't a name for it then. And for Hilary's family, there was no theory behind what they did, and they felt just as surprised by the process as the rest of us did. I'm not sure they fully understand what a gift that process was to everyone, but they are very excited about and interested in what's going on at Fairfax Hospital with our trauma and secondary trauma program.

From a trauma mastery aspect, I certainly think it's good for me to be doing this work, as well as for the people I'm working with. I don't need to tell anyone I'm working with that this happened to me. I know for myself that it will always have a 24 hours a day, seven days a week connection for me. It doesn't feel like work, what I do. It's not like me to say it's a calling, but when you have had your own connecting-the-dots experience, it definitely makes the field much more compelling. I have to be a part of it, it is so much fun for me. You know when you've been born again, you want everyone else to be born again. When you have the good fortune of something positive coming out of a tragedy, and when you believe it's possible for others to heal in this way, you want them to have this opportunity. In that way it is a trauma mastery thing for me.

Regarding how this work takes a toll on me, I feel like it takes no toll on me. I feel like it energizes me. I have figured out a plan for how much time I see direct trauma. I have an à la carte experience so that I don't put myself at the risk of compassion fatigue. I rotate from being in the ER and seeing horrible things to working with people on the floor who are bouncing back and experiencing their resiliency and then to working with people who months and years post-injury come to us because they are very curious about how they are going to grow from this. They have self-selected to come and figure out how to move away from what is hard and be in a different place in their lives, and you can't help but be completely inspired by those people.

My kids would say I'm totally neurotic about head injuries and that I'm overprotective, not effectively overprotective, as they continue to live their lives the way they want to, but I'm just more anxious. I'm very focused on prevention, because I'd say 98 percent of what I see in the ER could have been prevented if someone in the mix had done something different. I can see all the things that my now-teenage boys do as a potential injury. They would say, "She's over-the-top protective, she's really crazy." They don't follow my desires and they keep climbing trees and they don't always wear their helmets when they go biking, and it's just their luck that they haven't ended up in the ER. I think my husband would say that he thinks I have a really easy job because I portray it as really easy. He would say the way I've set it up is a piece of cake, so I'm pretty cheerful and it makes me happy to go. That is the much bigger tragedy to me, that you could live your life thinking that this is a chore and not recognizing that you have a choice. So many people live their lives that way. I have all my cycles, that's for sure, but it's not like I cycle into depression because of my job.

As far as taking care of myself, I do a lot of self-pampering. I exercise a lot, and one of the reasons I do is because when I'm exercising, I have no brain work going on, and that definitely resets me. Nothing goes through my brain. That is my meditation and my way to get centered. I think that when I am exercising I am more in touch with a sense of "This is me, and that's them." Even if I'm not conscious of it, I think that's largely what I'm doing. Even though I'm not aware of processing my work, I'm sure I'm passively processing somehow. With the kind of exercise that I tend to do, my aerobic capacity is so maxed that my brain just can't work, and I'm in the zone. If I'm running with someone, then I'm socializing at the same time. I'm at high risk of being somewhat depressed if I'm not exercising at an insane level.

I also have a fairly overdeveloped sense of denial. I'm able to be pretty separate from my work, and I don't do a lot of replaying of the traumas I see. Occasionally I think about them a lot, but I don't overexpose myself. I do know plenty of social workers who are overexposed, and they don't release that exposure, and they are not very happy people. If I didn't have this, I'd be locked up or my husband would be. I also have a great place to come home to, and I have a lot of my own time. I cook, I get massages, I do creative projects. I'm very protective of time that is just for me, and it happens to be feasible for me right now as I'm currently in a couple-year phase of having a lot of personal time. My kids are older now and my job is flexible. I have not always been this balanced. I was not quite as cheerful a person when the only time I could consider as my time was 30 minutes a day at the most. Now that I'm not raising my kids as much, I covet my time a lot more, and I work really hard to put those things in my day that I love to do. It's possible that it took a long time for me to figure this balance out. I wish I could have figured it out earlier, because then my children would have benefited from having a happier mother.

I believe that part of the reason why we were all able to heal as we did from Hilary's death has to do with the nurture. We were already a part of healthy community, and we had good social structures and communication in place, so we had a lot to work with. Surely our dispositions contributed to how we all ended up, too, but we're all really very different people. I'm working from the belief, then, that if we beef up the environment, and if we really pay attention to how trauma is handled, then the environment can handle whatever we bring to it. It has so much to do with how we manage the trauma. If we could have public systems set up and have some structure available for people, this would make a huge difference, because most families aren't going to have this set up already.

What I'm most excited about with our program, and what is fun for me, is the work that I do with the providers and former trauma patients. We take our trauma patients out of the patient role and put them in the educator role, in the role of expert, and have them talk to all kinds of medical providers as well as fire and rescue about what their experiences were like. Through this process they are able to transform the way they see themselves, as well as experience the gratification of being listened to by service providers. This is very connected to what I've learned in my own development, and to me it's some of the most exciting work we do.

When you bring both trauma survivors and service providers to the table and give them the tools to talk about what has happened, in a brief hour you can get a lot out of it. One of the most powerful aspects is that the paramedics and firefighters and other providers are able to see the parallels between the survivors' experiences and their own experiences. They are able to hear the survivors talk about the impact trauma has on their lives and their families, and whereas before, the providers may have felt it would be too much or too hard to recognize how they, themselves, are impacted by trauma exposure, when they hear the survivors share their stories, they can see how their experiences are so very similar. This experience and the awareness gained then opens up the possibility for the providers themselves to think, "Hey, maybe I can deal with this differently."

Another very exciting piece of this is that, when providers realize how much impact their work has on others, it helps them to feel unburdened. They see that they can make a difference. They hear directly from the trauma survivors how important it is. They really get that it matters how

> well they take care of themselves, and it matters how well they do their work.

Practicing Compassion for Myself and Others

> If your compassion does not include yourself, it is incomplete.
> Jack Kornfield, American Buddhist monk and educator

As we soak up the benefits of a microculture that is both loving and willing to hold us accountable, we are experiencing compassion in action. As obvious as this may seem, it may be helpful to remember and use as a model. Many people may have difficulty imagining what compassion for themselves might look like, and at times it may feel almost impossible to imagine practicing compassion toward those whose views are starkly at odds with our own. (Figure 10.2)

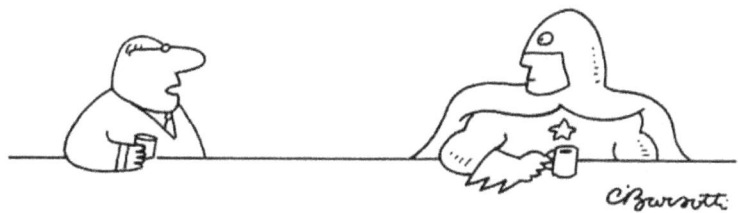

Figure 10.2: "Some of us are unsung heroes."

Nevertheless, maintaining and cultivating compassion for oneself and for others is a necessary part of trauma stewardship. It keeps us connected to our most loving values, from which our best selves can shine through. Qigong, which is said to be the most ancient of Eastern healing systems, sets forth the primary intention to transform all thoughts, feelings, and experiences into compassion. Compassion is connected to humility, to recognizing the ways in which we are both powerful and vulnerable, and to understanding how we are interdependent with one another.

For most of us, it is easiest to access compassion when we perceive no threat to ourselves. We can really feel for that dog with a broken leg or a friend who lost her job or the victims of flooding in India. But where does our compassion go when our boss yells at us? When a family blames us for the death of their loved one? When a government official lies to us?

When I talk about compassion in those circumstances, I am not talking about condoning others' behavior or having low expectations of ourselves and others. Rather, I am evoking the spirit of the Sufi wisdom that says, "Overcome any bitterness that may have come because you were not up to the magnitude of the pain that was entrusted to you." Throughout my experiences in life, personal and professional, I have found that meeting another's struggle with compassion, instead of getting our back up, decreases the suffering of all involved. We must understand that when humans act in damaging, unethical, harmful, or heinous ways, they are suffering enormous destruction internally. And so, instead of responding to conflicts as I previously did, by thinking, "Oh you did NOT just go there" and—figuratively—taking off my earrings for a fight, I try to call up the Dalai

Lama's request of us: Practice internal disarmament.

As both Pema Chödrön and bell hooks, an American author and social activist who focuses on the roles of race, class, and gender in systems of oppression, have written, sometimes compassion may mean taking firm or even severe steps. Acts of fierce compassion can range anywhere from reporting unethical behavior in your boss to demanding that a colleague seek drug treatment. The force behind such compassion is never self-righteousness. Our intentions are based in humility and knowing that we're in no way beyond reproach ourselves, even if our own shortcomings fall at a different place along the continuum. Our compassion comes from a desire to do no harm and have no harm done, not from a place of blaming and judgment. We're not thinking, "I'm good over here, but you're jacked up over there." When I am most challenged in this area, and find myself at a loss with a person or situation, I ask myself: "Have I ever knowingly or unknowingly caused suffering of another living being or of this planet?" Immediately I am overcome with how often I have—I can start with the half-dozen things I did this morning even before getting my children off to school. When I get to this place, I can exhale, and I'll often drop into repeating this version of the buddhist loving-kindness meditation:

> May I be free of suffering and the roots of suffering.
> May you be free of suffering and the roots of suffering.
> May we be free of suffering and the roots of suffering.
> May I find peace and the roots of peace.
> May you find peace and the roots of peace.
> May we find peace and the roots of peace.
> May I find joy and the roots of joy.
> May you find joy and the roots of joy.
> May we find joy and the roots of joy.
> May I find wellness and the roots of wellness.

May you find wellness and the roots of wellness.
May we find wellness and the roots of wellness.
May I be free.
May you be free.
May we be free.

We are powerful people, and what we contribute to the world has profound ramifications. The world does not need more hostility; it does not need more judgment; it does not need more walls between people, species, or nations. And so we can always contribute to the betterment of the world if we initiate compassionate action in the face of wrongdoing. We remember that we are fundamentally connected to this earth and its life, whatever the circumstances. As Chief Sealth, leader of the Suquamish and Duwamish tribes, said in 1854, we are all part of the same "web of life."

I've deepened my compassion so as to keep from numbing. I just try to look at every person as an individual and within a larger context of generational trauma, and it helps me connect. I'm grateful for that deeper compassion. It keeps me feeling.

Indian child welfare services social worker

If we are able to be compassionate toward those we passionately disagree with, we can be incredible students throughout our lifetime. We will greet each mistake or hardship we encounter as an opportunity to learn, and we will understand that we can learn just as much from another's path as our own. Since we know firsthand what it's like to fall down and slowly get back up, we can easily extend our compassion to others who do the same. Compassion provides us the breathing room we need to keep on keeping on. It also allows us to evolve: When we lack compassion, we become significantly stifled in our ability to connect with ourselves, with others, and with our lives.

The Buddha says, "When one is about to admonish another, there are five qualities to attend to. In due season will I speak, not out of season. In truth will I speak, not in falsehood.

Gently will I speak, not harshly. To their profit will I speak, not to their loss. With kindly intent or with compassion will I speak."

TRY THIS

1. Think of someone from early in your life who showed you a great deal of compassion. Hold them in your thoughts for a moment while you allow yourself to remember what it felt like to be in their presence.
2. Recall a time when you were particularly hard on yourself. Ask yourself what your deepest fear was at that time. Close your eyes and replay the situation in your mind, imagining how you could have responded to yourself more compassionately. Notice how this shift in response feels.
3. Generate a list of six people or situations in your life where you think an increase in your compassion could significantly alter the dynamic. Make an intention to approach one of these

people/situations with increased compassion each month for six months. Pay attention to the difference in your life.

What Can I Do for Large-Scale Systemic Change?

When I'm not at work, I focus on the cohousing community where I live. It really helps me to remember that while I am surrounded by so much pain in my work, I am also a part of something larger. I am a part of a larger movement of socially and ecologically conscious people who are thinking about how we live, and for me, it makes all the difference.
Public health worker

For some people, the internal focus of a daily practice may at first seem like a distraction, another excuse to privilege individual self-absorption over a collective push for global social change. As it happens, the opposite is true. Buddhist teachers often talk about compassion as moving in an ever-widening circle. We start with ourselves, and then extend our compassion to those who are close to us, and finally extend it to people all over the world. The deeper our compassion, the clearer our sense of how we can take action is likely to be.

In every trauma stewardship workshop I facilitate, participants ask me, "What can I do to change the systems I work in?" The "system" may be a small rural health clinic, the environmental movement, or perhaps the Democratic Party. As I begin my response, I often remind my colleagues that we may unknowingly influence systems simply by altering the way we interact with them. We must never underestimate the power of changing ourselves, of committing to being a force for liberation, light, wellness, justice, and right action wherever we go. On one level, this is the only thing we can ever really control—ourselves.

That said, *if* we have energy, *if* we are inspired, and *if* we feel that we can interact with larger systems while preserving our integrity and a healthy and hopeful sense of self, then we have the choice to support transformation on a larger scale. It is my experience personally and professionally that the most difficult tasks for individuals lie not in high-profile, macro efforts to shift something externally, but rather in the smaller moments of moderating our own behavior: letting someone merge in front of us on the freeway, being meticulous with our way of talking to loved ones, reaching out to a neighbor who belongs to a different political party, forgiving someone we feel has done us wrong. It takes great commitment to bring this level of mindfulness and compassion to large-scale reform—but if we are to create change with integrity, we must be willing to question our actions. As Archbishop Desmond Tutu says, "Our means must be consistent with our ends." (Figure 10.3)

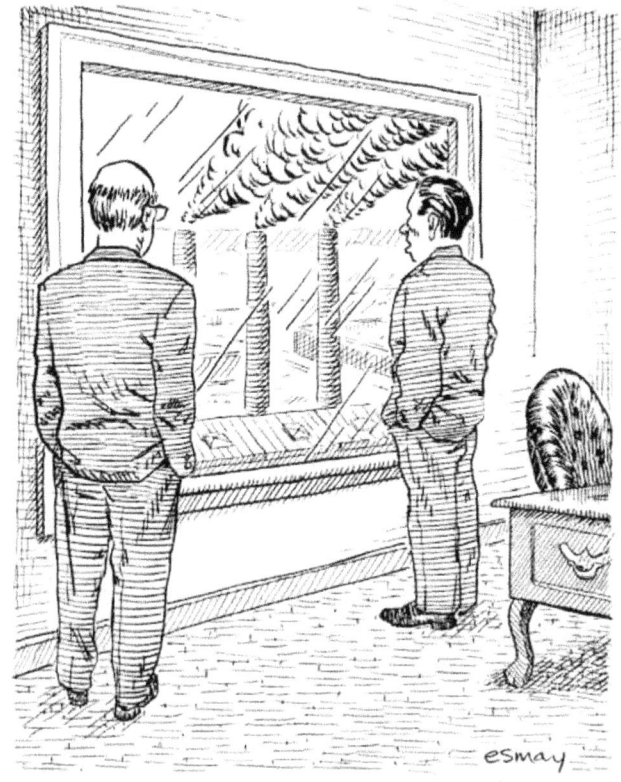

Figure 10.3: "Can't we just dye the smoke green?"

For those who can enter into large-scale reform with their wits about them, how to go about it? Behaviors that are meant to serve others eventually emerge as a natural element of any mindfulness practice. As Connie Burk has said, "Because we are agents who benefit from and are enfranchised to create the political, economic, and material conditions of the actual external world, we are responsible for it. We are responsible for and implicated in and obligated to its transformation."

For some people, taking responsibility means not gossiping in the workplace; for others it means boycotting a certain shoemaker. Some people volunteer weekly in inner-city after-school programs; others go into politics. Almost without thinking, we may translate our compassion into action.

Jill Robinson founded Animals Asia, an animal welfare organization that operates in six countries. She says, "Over the years of working on animal welfare issues in Asia, I have become a more serious and more focused person, but I am by nature an optimist. This has enabled me to keep on track when we see such utter devastation to animals during the course of our work. I personally use these visions of horror towards creating change. This may take the form of simply purging in writing—almost channeling those animals in essays that hopefully will reach the hearts of decision makers, of the media, or our supporters. Progress is a driving force—it is empowering and addictive as we see the fruits of our work translate into solid help for the animals of Asia. Of course, the most positive impact is not only seeing the progress in our work and goals, but being with animals that have so completely put their misery behind. They teach us, heal us, and rescue us as surely as we rescue them. If I have a hard day, for example, I'll smile and talk into the walkie-talkie telling the team I'm off to have a meeting with Jasper ('my' bear). Many of my colleagues do the same with 'their' bears."

Marianne Knuth founded Kufunda, a learning village in Zimbabwe. Its purpose is to "inspire the co-creation of strong, life-affirming communities in Zimbabwe and beyond by living and sharing the wisdom, practices, and social systems that are required for such communities." While Zimbabwe remains enveloped in a socioeconomic crisis, Knuth believes that "the beginning is to support people to reclaim their sense of wealth and wisdom. Great energy is released when we stop focusing on what we don't have, and when we begin to pay attention to what we do have and build on this with each other in innovative and creative ways." As the Arundhati Roy quote featured on the Kufunda Web site says, "Another world is not only possible. She is on the way."

Cameron Sinclair and Kate Stohr founded Architecture for Humanity, whose mission is to "promote architectural and design solutions to global, social and humanitarian crises." They have lived and worked in some of the most devastated places in the world. Every day, they face people in desperate need of shelter. Yet they remain hopeful, inspired by an unwavering conviction that "where resources and expertise are scarce, innovative, sustainable and collaborative design can make a difference." There is no end to the myriad ways to be engaged in repairing the world, or *tikkun olam,* as it is called in the Jewish tradition.

TRY THIS

1. Think of an area in your life where you are part of the dominant group (race, class, sexual identity, or another area). Generate a list of four ways that you could be an ally to someone. Dedicate one action per week to using your privilege for good. For example, if you are a U.S. citizen, research a group working for the rights of immigrants and refugees and see how you may be able to lend a hand.
2. Identify a system you are involved in, and think of three ways you could work toward positive change in that system. Remember that you must avoid any approach that will leave you feeling more bitter, more jaded, or more isolated.
3. Develop a relationship with someone in leadership and do something once a month to provide direct support to the person, whether you share a meal, offer to shoulder some of his/her workload, or arrange for him/her to get an acupuncture session. You might

choose the director of a nonprofit, a principal of a nearby elementary school, or an elected official. Remember how often leadership is isolated, unsupported, and set up for failure. Through reaching out, you are making every effort to keep your leaders as tethered and grounded as possible.

A DREAM REALIZED POLLY HALFKENNY

PITTSBURGH, PENNSYLVANIA

Polly Halfkenny began to be politically active as an undergraduate student and became a mother while going to school full time. Figuring out how to combine family, work, and politics began early for her. She was an activist engaged in the antiwar, civil rights, and anti-repression movements in the 1960s and early 1970s, participating in the Northern Student Movement and Freedom Stayouts, the Committee to Free Angela Davis, and the National Alliance Against Racist and Political Repression. She also worked full time and returned to graduate school to get a master's in special education in 1969. In 1967, she joined the Communist Party, of which she was a member until 1991, when she joined the Committees of Correspondence for Democracy and Socialism (CCDS), which was formed by many who left the Communist Party in the United States and other Marxists or Democratic Socialists. Most of her jobs throughout her career have combined politics and work: urban planning, education, child advocacy, policy analysis, and child therapy.

Often the work I was involved in was dealing with immediate repression that people faced, including our family. We were living in a low-income family housing development and there were real issues going on, including police repression and racist reactions to the desegregation of Boston public schools. My children were going to public school; as a biracial family we faced racist violence as well as reactions within the African-American community to attacks by whites. The Communist

Party was essential for me because I was looking for an organization that put all these pieces that I was dealing with in some context as well as a larger framework, and something that said that what we need is systemic change. A lot of the debate about what to do was going on in the student movements and in antiwar and community organizations. The Party enabled me to think about how all these elements we were facing fit in the big picture, how can we deal with these things day to day, and how can we make systemic change.

If you ask my children, I'm not sure they would agree that I balanced or maintained activism in a way that was manageable. I think they often felt that politics took me away from home too much. There was a point in time when I really cut back on political work, as the children got older. I cut back on meetings, although I don't think they perceived that I did. I've learned since to appreciate that their perception is their reality. That's what you have to deal with. Not your perceptions of their reality, but the perception from their point of view and its impact on their lives.

I came from a very small town with a 1950s education, so my going to college was an education in terms of skills, being in an urban environment, and being amidst political change. There were tremendous ideological debates going on in that time. I was hungry for political and intellectual dialogue and debate, and I sort of walked into the middle of this and I thought, "This is heaven." That was finding a home for myself. I was no longer the oddball reading beat poetry under my covers in a small community. I had walked into a school where there was this lively debate going on, and I thought, "This is what my life is about!" I felt like I had found it, and it was about a bigger picture.

Part of what was very helpful for me in trying to make things manageable and one of the things that came out of that period of time is that I've always been a part of collectives. I've always had very good friends who have been a part of helping me provide. It wasn't just that they supported me, but that they tried to help the reality of a person who was an activist and had responsibility to a family, especially during a time when I was single parenting, which made it much, much more difficult. So things like their trying to organize events that involved children, for example. I grew up in a big family, which may have helped me with the cooperation and working-well-together piece, too.

Other things that were helpful included having a wonderful therapist who helped me to figure out how to do what I was trying to do. I was active in the women's movement and I have a lot of friends. I have a great deal of difficulty asking for help, but I'm smart enough to have friends who will ask if they can help me with something. The political organizations I was a part of gave me confidence. One of the things that changed dramatically from the time I was first involved is how the movement viewed women. The changes and growth within the Party in terms of political and theoretical education eventually led to a commitment that women should be in leadership. If you're relegated to the mimeograph machine and there's not a commitment to fighting racism and sexism in the group, then it's very debilitating. I've always been a part of organizations that had a class analysis and a commitment to fight racism and sexism. Having people I could talk to and who I could really connect with was helpful—and still is.

One of the most basic defenses is denial, so I never ever stopped to think about how difficult it was to be a single parent until it was done. My mother really was a feminist in her own way. I grew up with this idea, watching her, that you sew your kids' clothes, you make their Halloween costumes, you make your own holiday presents, you make their lunches each day before school. That was my expectation of what a mom is. By conscious choice, we didn't have a television, so after the kids go to bed, you knit or crochet or do these types of projects.

What helped me to keep going is that I really believe in the goodness of human beings and that people can change. I have this capacity to get up in the morning and look at the sunshine and say, "Hey, what are we going to do today?" There are always people around me who have this same kind of optimism and belief that another world is possible, and I draw from them. The communities we create help not only in the day-to-day stuff but also in holding these larger beliefs.

When my children were in junior high and high school, I was active in the trade union movement (Local 509 SEIU). I was also active in local town politics while I worked for the commonwealth at what was then the Office for Children. I left that job because I was going to be laid off and the timing was good for me to think about how to best do what I wanted—how did I want to live the rest of my life given my split from the Communist Party and my need to rethink priorities, analysis, what is socialism/communism, democracy, and so on. I was also asking myself, "How do I find a different political home?" because the Party had been a home for me. I left the Office for Children in the fall of 1992 and immediately started law school when my youngest graduated from high school. I became a labor lawyer upon graduating, working for the United Electrical, Radio and Machine Workers of America (UE), of which I am now general counsel. The UE can best be described as a national, independent, rank and file, democratic trade union, not affiliated with either the AFL-CIO or CTW. In my current work, I'm able to combine all of those things that are priorities for me, including politics, and I see this union as a part of making systemic change in the country.

But it's really not simple. I don't want it ever to be seen that you can't do both or that you have to make choices that make people feel that their lives are in conflict with their politics. I was fortunate that I was able to have access to education in a way that did not incur debt; I could have professional, nonprofit-advocacy-type jobs that paid enough that you feel like you're doing good work and you're able to support your family. In essence, I think you have to both confront immediate manifestations of injustice and work for systemic change. That is what I did. I fought oppression where I was at the same time that I fought for a long-term vision related to fundamental change in economic, social, and power relationships in the U.S.—while raising two children (mostly as a single parent) and working full time or part time all the while.

If all you do is the day-to-day stuff and you don't figure out where you're going in the big picture, you can burn out pretty easily. On the other hand, if you're an armchair revolutionary, what's that worth?

CHAPTER ELEVEN

WEST • Finding Balance

Coming full circle into the west, we call upon the strength and introspection of the air element. By striving to achieve balance in our lives, moving energy through, and reminding ourselves of all that we are grateful for, we attend to needs as basic as the air we breathe. We celebrate the strength we receive by connecting to our inner self through our breath. The air is seen as universal power in traditional cultures; when we honor the changing winds, we see the impermanence of everything and understand the beauty of being awake for the here and now.

Engaging with Our Lives Outside of Work

I didn't realize how bad I'd gotten until I left.

Health care worker

For many of us committed to the "repair of the world," it can be a desperate struggle to find a balance between our selves and our work. On one hand, it can be tempting to harden ourselves and disassociate from our work when it gets difficult. On the other, we get buried so deeply in the brutality around us that we forget to take care of ourselves entirely. Either way, it may become increasingly difficult to feel whole again. For this reason, it is important to create a work environment for yourself that is as humane as possible.

I was heartened to learn that some child protective services workers in Seattle meet in the local park to practice tae kwon do during their lunch hour, and that others drive down to the lake and sit eating their lunches with a view of the Cascade Mountains. A domestic violence advocate particularly endeared herself to me by describing the five-minute lunch breaks she took in the always-hectic emergency shelter where she worked. She would close her door and spread out a white paper napkin on her desk, arrange her modest meal on her makeshift placemat, and, to the best of her ability, eat her food in relative peace and quiet. Meanwhile, other workers struggle to avoid car accidents while eating their lunches and driving between home visits or meetings. Some people don't go to the bathroom for the whole time they're at work, and others work when they are sick. In New Orleans, one dedicated nurse continued to volunteer at a clinic even while she had mono. These types of stories are not unusual. (Figure 11.1)

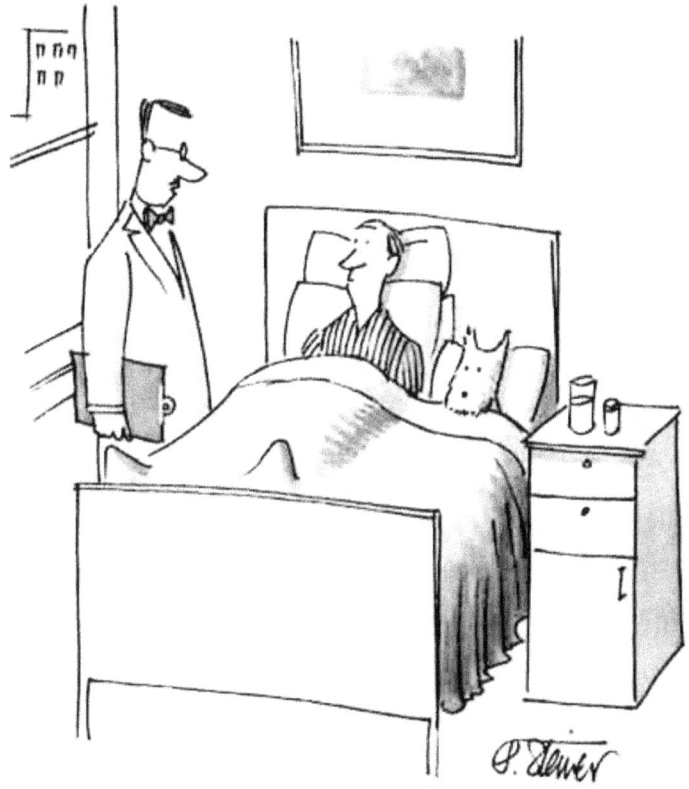

Figure 11.1: "Under our holistic approach, Mr. Wyndot. we not only treat your symptoms, we also treat your dog."

In the long term, as we've seen, it simply doesn't work to check our true selves at the door and hope that we can reconnect at the end of the day. Whatever we can do right now to create a more holistic or integrated approach to our work is a worthwhile effort. Consider your particular work environment and daily routine. What moments can you reclaim to attend to your inner well-being? Three minutes between meetings? Part of the drive to a site visit? The five minutes you have when a patient is late? Any one of these may be an opportunity to regroup and center yourself.

For years, I was blessed to have a beloved rottweiler named Caleb in my life. He eventually led me to the field of animal-assisted therapy. But before I even knew such a field existed, I watched in amazement as my dog connected with individuals and groups in crisis or transition or in pain. Caleb would find that one person in a domestic violence support group who most needed to connect with unconditional acceptance. He would move slowly toward her, placing his huge head gently on her leg, and she would gratefully stroke his fur for the duration of the group. Caleb would lean into the tattooed, pierced, and emaciated body of a distraught homeless youth who hadn't talked to anyone in weeks, and the boy would crouch down and hug him. Caleb could sense which child in an AIDS support group was most afraid of him and of life in general. He would wind his way around the group until he reached her. He would place himself flat on the floor, making his 110-pound self seem as small as possible. Finally the child would reach out, taking one of his ears in her small hand—she would pet first one ear, then the other, and then his whole head, for the remainder of the hour. (Figure 11.2)

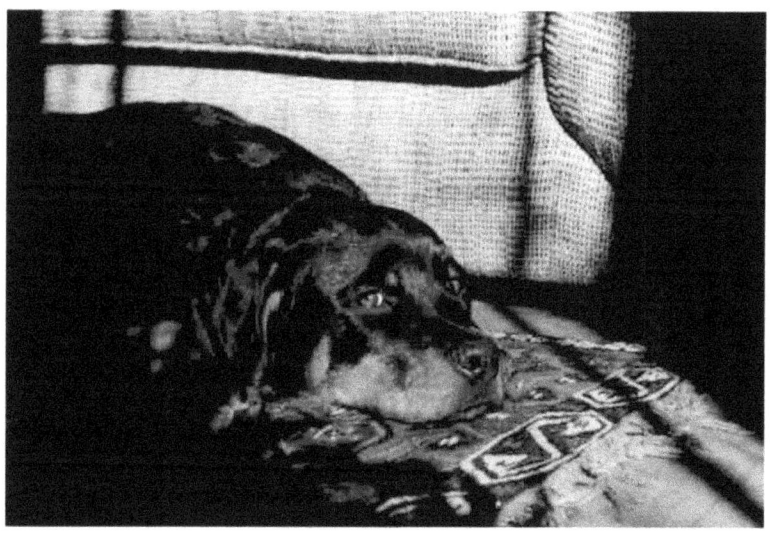

Figure 11.2

I was able to do work during that time of my life in a way I never could have without Caleb. He was so frequently able to bridge what is often a large chasm between humans. Equally important, he provided a foundation of comfort and inspiration for me. How depressed could I get with my soul mate by my side at all times?

It is also a very good plan every now and then to go away and have a little relaxation, for when you come back to the work, your judgment will be surer, since to remain constantly at work will cause you to lose the power of judgment. It is also advisable to go some distance away, because then the work appears smaller, and more of it is taken in at a glance, and a lack of harmony or proportion in the various parts and the colors of the objects is more readily seen.

Leonardo da Vinci, Italian engineer and painter (Figure 11.3)

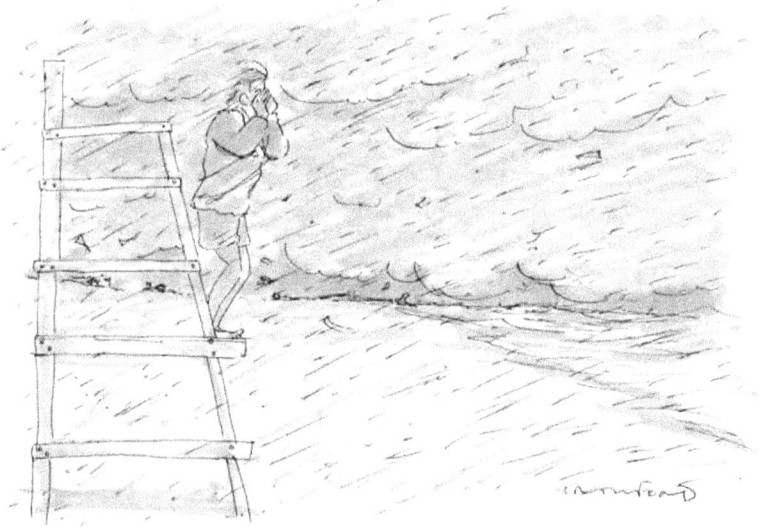

Figure 11.3: "I said, 'I'm not on duty! I just came back to get my flip-flops.'"

Never underestimate what you can weave into your shift, work, or career to make it a healthier place for you to be. Decide that being a martyr in the workplace is a thing of the past. Negotiate a sane schedule before accepting a job, and renegotiate your current agreement if need be. Surround yourself with colleagues who will support you as you stick to your agreed-upon hours and take time off. Be a positive force in your workplace: When your colleagues leave for vacation, tell them to enjoy themselves and not to look back; remind them that you have everything handled. Don't perpetuate the guilt-tripping that so often goes on, with muttered comments like, "It must be nice for you. Wish we could all take time away." Remember that we are only a benefit to those we serve if we are able to have some true balance in our life. As is written in the Daily Tao, "The sun shines half a day, the moon dominates the rest. Even contemplation should have its proper duration." When you go away from work, really leave. No pagers, cell phones, or devices you have to check. Really engaging in the rejuvenating activities of your life outside of work is essential for trauma stewardship. As one health care worker said, "I make an appointment with sleep."

> My children recently asked me if I could remember the last time we spent time together, all of us, as a family. It's been so long, I can't even remember the last time.
> Wildlife conservationist, Democratic Republic of Congo

TRY THIS

1. Identify one thing that you would love to incorporate into your workday but are certain you could not. Now try everything in your power to make that aspiration a reality.
2. Write down all your sick leave time, vacation time, and mental health days. Start planning ahead ... now!
3. Remember that the labor movement and countless other individuals worked hard to create weekends and breaks and more humane working conditions. Resolve to honor those who have gone before you by agreeing only to a sustainable work schedule and sticking to it.

Moving Energy Through

> I haven't breathed since last week.
>
> Community-clinic executive director during a crisis period

We can strive for balance in other ways, too. We can't get mired in one overstressed state. We need to keep our internal energy moving, like the wind.

In traditional Chinese medicine, there is a belief that dis-ease in one's being comes in part from stagnant energy. When we talk about energy, we are talking about your life force, your vitality, what it is that makes you *you,* your very essence. It's what gets you up in the morning, what you feel when someone walks into the room, the sensations you recall when you think about a person or animal who has died. An important part of well-being in this tradition is keeping the energy moving and not allowing it to stagnate around any one feeling or issue. This is an invaluable practice for those of us who interact with suffering: being able to exist with awareness amid radiating waves of pain. Rather than absorbing and accumulating them, we can learn to let them ripple out and away.

Peter Levine invites us to learn from animals in the wild to gain insight into why, as humans, we are so often traumatized, while animals so rarely are. Through his decades of study, he found that humans and animals have in common three basic responses to threat, each of them directed by the primitive, reptilian part of the brain. These are the flight, fight, and immobility (freezing) responses.

When we perceive a threat, a great deal of energy is summoned. When we are able to fight or flee, that energy is naturally discharged—and as we see with animals in the wild, it is possible to return to life as it was before the threat. If we are unable to fight or flee from a threat, our organism instinctively constricts (or freezes) in a last-ditch effort at self-preservation. Again, when an animal in the wild survives danger through immobility, it will unfreeze itself, literally shake off the accumulated energy, and continue to graze or care for its young—in other words, it will generally go about its business.

As Levine found, however, this release is not so easy for humans. When we move into the constricted freezing response, a tremendous amount of energy becomes bound up and begins to overwhelm our nervous system. If our reptilian brain impulses were allowed to run their course, we would discharge this expanse of highly charged energy once the threat passed. Instead, however, our highly evolved neocortex (rational brain) often gets in the way. The fear and desire for control that arise in the neocortex can be so powerful that they interrupt the restorative impulses that would allow for a necessary form of discharge. As humans, then, we are stranded partway through the same nervous system cycle that keeps animals well and thriving. In us, undischarged residual energy becomes the seed for deep-rooted trauma. Many of the symptoms of trauma exposure response we discussed in chapter 4 are signs of our organism's effort to contain this undischarged energy.

As Levine sums it up in *Waking the Tiger*, "The neocortex is not powerful enough to override the instinctual defense response to threat and danger—the fight, flee, or freeze response. In this respect we humans are still inextricably bound to our animal heritage. Animals, however, do not have a highly evolved neocortex to interfere with the natural return to normal functioning through some form of discharge. In humans, trauma occurs as a result of the initiation of an instinctual cycle that is not allowed to finish."

Levine has used his research as the basis for an approach to healing trauma that he calls "somatic experiencing." Practitioners of somatic experiencing believe that "the core of traumatic reaction is ultimately physiological, and it is at this level that healing begins." Levine's method applies a variety of techniques to liberate energy that has become frozen as a result of trauma. When it succeeds, the nervous system is able to return to its original resilient and self-regulating state.

Learning how to work with our internal energies is one of the first steps in supporting our body's innate capacity to heal. We can gently explore ways to keep our internal energy flowing. When it is blocked, we can look for activities that unblock it. This will create the foundation we need for long-term wellness.

It's like I feel all this toxicity build up inside of me, and if I don't go surfing or go biking or go for a run, I can't function anymore.
Mark Thanassi, attending physician, emergency medicine, Santa Clara, California

In Jewish tradition there is the practice of sitting shiva when someone dies. For the vast majority of Jews, support for the bereaved during this time takes the form of intimate contact and conversation. In some Orthodox communities, however, one of the guidelines for sitting shiva is that the visitors are expected to talk with the mourners only once they have been explicitly addressed by the bereaved. One reason for this is a respect for the enormous power of bearing witness. It's not about what we do, what we say, or how we touch—it's about being present in a way that tells those who are suffering that they are not and never will be alone. Because we are all inherently connected, the witnesses will share some of the burden of what the mourners are experiencing—even if they do no other thing.

If we are to remain physically, emotionally, and spiritually healthy, however, sharing the pain cannot translate into soaking it all up. The energy of pain must be kept moving. If all the struggle and hardship we witness accumulates and takes root, it will grow so large that any light we have within us will be obscured. Uprooting this accumulated anguish is much, much harder than preventing it from taking root in the first place. Jack Kornfield says, "What has been entrusted to us, and what do we do with it? It's simple. When we possess [others' sufferings] in an unhealthy way, we worry, we're caught, and we're neither at peace nor free. Since it all changes, it's guaranteed that it's going to change, we need to discover a capacity to let go, a graciousness of heart."

For many of us, this concept may require some radical reframing. Letting go may sound like being passive or going limp. The thought of relaxing our grip may fill us with fear. You may be someone who was raised to believe that action=movement=growth=survival, and so when you think of stillness, you may come up with the equation stillness=surrender=powerlessness=death. Although eventually you may want to question these associations, it is not necessary to abandon them overnight. We are talking about moving energy not necessarily through stillness per se but through a mindful and disciplined approach of detoxing, cleansing, and putting our burdens down. Some can do this using rapid actions such as running, while others move toward the equation of stillness=awareness=connection=action=life. Those people may practice focused breathing, meditating, walking, gardening, chanting, and so on. As Thich Nhat Hanh said to a student who asked just how much she needed to slow down, "You never see us monks running. We walk slowly. It's too hard to be present when you're moving quickly."

So we talk about moving energy through as a way to keep ourselves at our optimal level. One way to move energy through is by conscious breathing. It may come as a surprise to many of us that attention to the breath is central to keeping ourselves in a state of balance, yet every ancient tradition has as a critical element mindful and deliberate breathing. Native Americans have held Sun Dancing and sweat lodge Ceremonies for centuries; Tarahumara Indians have run as a tenet central to their well-being; East Indian traditions have practiced yoga since the beginning of recorded time and, more recently, have held focused-laughter gatherings. Meditative traditions all over the world have developed techniques that sharpen the mind's awareness and cultivate insight using one's own breath as the primary guide. Breathing is the one regular, life-sustaining process we can always observe within ourselves. It is evidence of the present moment rising and passing away. It is a constant reminder that everything, including our own lives, is subject to a universal law, the law of impermanence. This perspective can free us to realize the myriad choices we have to live harmoniously, with deeper awareness, in this life.

> The ordinary response to atrocities is to banish them from consciousness. Certain violations of the social compact are too terrible to utter aloud.... Atrocities, however, refuse to be buried. Equally as powerful as the desire to deny atrocities is the conviction that denial does not work. Folk wisdom is filled with ghosts who refuse to rest in their graves until their stories are told.
>
> Judith Herman, author of Trauma and Recovery and associate clinical professor of psychiatry at Harvard Medical School

When I was in New Orleans facilitating trauma stewardship workshops after Hurricane Katrina, I had the privilege of working with the People's Hurricane Relief Fund. Many of the city's residents had been left with a pained, hollow look in their eyes, but at the Relief Fund I met two women who stood out because of their radiance. Kimberley Richards and Kanika Taylor-Murphy are community organizers, activists, and educators. Neither was in New Orleans when the storm hit land and the levees broke. Both survived the trauma as first responders. One lost everything but her brick house in Picayune, Mississippi. Both continued to live with ample subsequent trauma exposure as they worked with the People's Hurricane Relief Fund and the People's Institute for Survival and Beyond, as well as other organizations, family members, and friends, in an effort to rebuild New Orleans.

I had the opportunity to inquire what they had done to care for themselves that was helpful. Kimberley Richards said, "For a month after the storm hit, I wasn't doing anything to take care of myself. And then I started getting sick, like in my head. Since then I have walked every morning for an hour or two. I'm joined by about seven other women now, and we walk through the neighborhoods and I breathe. It's hard because my oppression tells me if I have that time, I should be helping other people. My oppression tells me that if I'm up that early, I should be writing a grant. But I keep doing it, I keep walking." Kanika Taylor-Murphy said that practicing qigong and walking with Richards and their comrades were what allowed her to keep on keeping on.

Billie Lawson has spent her career on the front lines of trauma as well as immersed in trauma debriefings throughout the state of Washington. She creates cues throughout her day simply to remind herself to breathe deeply. Each time her phone rings at work, she takes a full inhale and exhale before she picks up the receiver. It's an exercise she gets to perform frequently!

Other ways of moving energy through include working out, writing, singing, chanting, dancing, martial arts, walking, and laughing, just as long as these activities are done with mindfulness. One colleague who works with bombing victims in northern Iraq as part of a Christian peacemaking effort said, "I like to do emptying exercises—meditation, deep breathing, touching nature, and thinking about how

I am not keeping or holding on to anything."

TRY THIS

1. Stand or sit in a comfortable position. As you raise your hands above your head, breathe in. As you lower your arms, breathe out. Do this 20 times, slowly.
2. Commit to walking or running or wheeling or biking outside for five minutes during every hour that you're working. During this five minutes, focus on breathing in deeply and breathing out slowly. Notice anything beautiful around you and breathe that in as well.
3. Initiate a co-counseling type of relationship with a colleague or friend whom you can call on regularly. Agree to counsel each other, if only for five minutes. Let your friend start the talking and listen attentively with a calming presence. Then it's your turn. Say whatever is in your heart and mind, moving it out of your system, while your partner in the exercise listens

attentively for five minutes. Repeat frequently.

WHY HUMOR HEATHER ANDERSEN

SEATTLE, WASHINGTON

CURRENTLY: Founder, HumanSource consulting; named plaintiff for marriage equality lawsuit (Andersen v. Washington State, 2006).

FORMERLY: Author of a dissertation on humor and leadership; Clinical director, Hospice of Seattle.

Humor has the ability to help you shift perspective quickly. It can be much like psychotherapy, only faster! Humor opens up some little door that lets you see yourself and the situation in a bigger picture. And sometimes it's that little door that can save your life.

I remember years ago I was very depressed with suicidal thoughts. I was on the freeway and I decided I just wanted to end it all then and there. I saw a huge truck coming up behind me, and I decided that I'm going to turn into it and let it kill me. Then I thought, maybe I should just look at the guy and see who I'm going to have take me out, you know, just connect for a second and look at him. I noticed, then, that the truck he was driving was a Darigold Dairy truck, and I thought, "Only you, Heather, would have something as wholesome as a milk truck take you out." And I started laughing, and it kept me from swerving in front of him, and I was able to reach my work, go inside, and call my therapist. As an adult, that was when humor literally saved my life.

Humor also cracks you open in a way so that you can be healed, too. I grew up in a crazy, chaotic household; humor was a way that I could move adroitly through it. I could protect myself with it. I could use it to fend off a parent's bad mood or a crazy situation. I could be the clown. I knew that if I could get my parents to laugh about something, then they would ease up.

When I was 15, I started working in a nursing home full time after school, and there humor was a psychological defense. We laughed so hard there, about so many things. I remember this one shift when I was cleaning up the body of an old gentleman after he had died, and this small TV was on across the room. I can still remember the Pepsi commercial that was on, with their theme song of "Come alive, you're in the Pepsi generation!" Seeing that dead body right in front of me and these young, healthy, come-alive-you're-in-the-Pepsi-generation people running in the background made me laugh out loud. I was able to see the juxtaposition and it was protective. It took me out of the moment and gave me the emotional and psychological distance I needed to deal with what was at hand, and to do my job well.

The in-group humor we'd do a lot of times. These are times when you take the power away from whatever psychological situation is threatening you and reduce it using humor. It is such a fine line to do it respectfully. The humor always needs to preserve the human dignity of the person and yourself. It's where you talk about one of your own foibles rather than about the patient. It can allow you to keep moving through, because while somewhere in your head you're saying, "This is psychologically stressful," you are also thinking, at that very moment, "I can hardly wait to tell them this at the morning break." That allows you to get through the next bit with that patient. It's like what the American author and radio personality Clifton Fadiman says about a sense of humor: "What is a sense of humor? Surely not the ability to understand a joke. It comes rather from a residing feeling of one's own absurdity. It is the ability to understand a joke—and that the joke is oneself."

It was a similar thing when my brother died. The funeral home staff was about to zip up the body bag, and I said, "Don't zip it up all the way," and my brother's wife then introduced her dead husband to the mortician. The humor I found in introducing a dead body to a mortician gave me enough distance so they could wheel him out of the house, and I was able to stay present with my family in a deeper way without being totally absorbed in the sadness of it all at that moment.

I have that comic vision—as the American psychologist and therapeutic humorist Steven Sultanoff describes it, "A way of perceiving the world that allows us to be receptive to the humor around and within us." I don't know if it was genetic or I developed it; I imagine it came from both the nature and nurture routes. But I do have it and it has been one of my greatest assets in life.

I remember when we were in the courtroom for the Supreme Court hearing on the marriage equality lawsuit, and it was so incredibly intense. I noticed that there were two men sitting behind us holding hands, and I thought to myself, "I didn't think they were gay." So I started eavesdropping, and they were praying that God would strike us down and that we would be taken to the fires of Hell! I almost laughed out loud thinking how the two men would react if they knew I interpreted their hand-holding as gay men there in support of us. That helped ease some tension for me; it got me out of myself and my ego so that I could see in some way the larger absurdity of it all.

I love to quote Leo Rosten, the Polish-born American educator and humorist: "[Humor is] the affectionate communication of insight." In my humor research with leaders, I found that there were leaders who felt "affectionately encountered" when I'd use humor with them. Most people in leadership positions, and I would say most of us in general, do not have a large repertoire of humor techniques—humor is an untapped resource. Many of the leaders in my study used negative humor—like sarcasm, which is more used for controlling others and drawing boundaries; or making fun of or shaming others. What's so important with humor is the intent and the feeling behind it. It's such a reflection of a person, in that you can tell so much about a person's values and psychological well-being by how well and how often they use humor. Some years ago, I was leading a grief group with a number of nurses who were working with families who had lost a child recently. Yet, somehow we were able to bring humor into the group, and the members were able to laugh a great deal despite all the tragedy they bore witness to. Eventually one of the supervisors overhearing the laughter coming from our conference room said, "That doesn't sound like a grief group to me. I'm not sure they still need to meet." Clearly she didn't understand the tie between grief and humor.

Humor gives me physical and psychological energy; as I have become more open and alive, my laugh has changed. I laugh really loud now, from deep in the belly, and that's a good thing. Physiologically that gives you an internal massage of your organs. It's absolutely part of my every day. Improvisation is such an important thing to be able to use as well. The big thing with improv is that you never refuse an offering. Through improv you're able to open to what is and work with what you're given. Watch people who use humor well; they are usually folks who say yes a lot to others and to life.

In my dissertation I created a model of humor use—the Andersen Humor Model. As part of it, I say that your use of humor has to match with you as a person (ego appropriate) and it has to fit the environment in which you're working (eco-appropriate). When you make a snappy rejoinder and you realize that it didn't align with your values, or you realize it was not the right time or right place, then apologize. You start being more aware and making sure your humor aligns, but you still continue to take risks. Simultaneously, we need to educate ourselves to be sure that our humor is not oppressive or offensive in any way. We all have a responsibility to stop oppression that is couched in humor, and people in leadership positions are responsible for making sure their policies reflect this.

Steven Sultanoff has some great articles where he writes about humor strengthening our physical and psychological immune systems. Biochemically we are affected by humor and the release of immunoglobulin when we laugh. Additionally, humor helps us regenerate our psychological immune system and helps us alter how we feel, think, and behave. One aspect he talks about, which I love, is in the humorist and cartoonist James Thurber's expression, "Humor is a kind of emotional chaos told about calmly and quietly in retrospect." Those moments of realizing "It wasn't funny at the time!" are an example of what Thurber and Sultanoff mean by that. While humor in no way reduces the seriousness of a traumatic situation, according to Sultanoff it can later "lighten the load of coping with trauma and aids in the healing process by offering perspective and assisting the client on the path towards recovery."

Margie Brown, a recognized teacher and artist in biblical humor in the U.S., describes humor this way: "Humor happens when two worlds collide. Something unexpected has to happen that jolts you up and out of the normal pattern, and then you start laughing. Humor is the synapse between the regular and the surprising. Every time we laugh, we are making a leap between two worlds."

Gratitude

> The air feels so nice right now, it just feels perfect.
>
> Hurricane Katrina survivor, after returning to New Orleans from her evacuation to Austin, Texas

One of the ways that we can consciously create a sense of balance in our lives is by cultivating our sense of gratitude. Locating something to be thankful for at all times is an essential part of trauma stewardship. It is yet another way that we can reframe our circumstances through mindfulness. Remind yourself that while the suffering may seem endless, so is what we have to be grateful for; it just might be less obvious and take a more creative approach to find it. An example of this is the practice of welcoming the difficult people in our lives as "teachers," which we discussed in chapter 8, as part of our investigation of trauma mastery. Viewing our most challenging relationships as our teachers can help make bleak times bearable. It also roots us in humility and graciousness, which is much better than arrogance and indignation. (Figure 11.4)

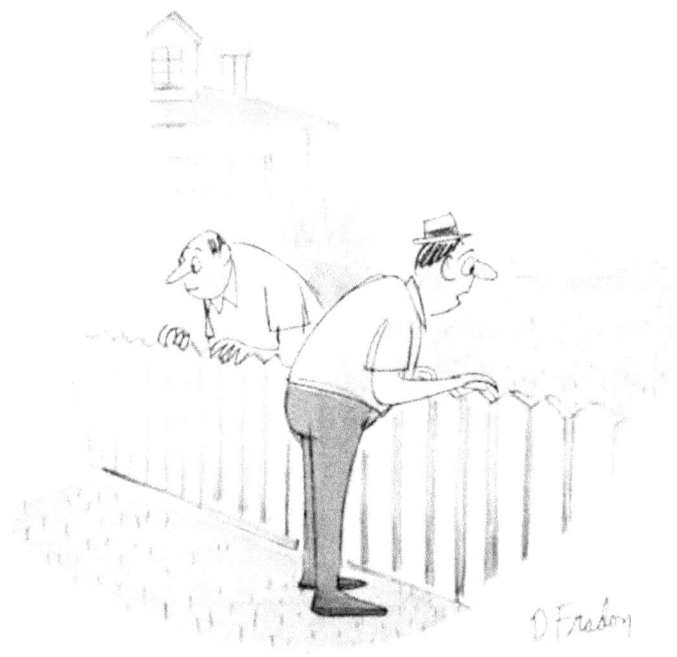

Figure 11.4: "I couldn't disagree with you more. I think yours is greener."

I encourage organizations to weave gratitude time into their staff meetings. After the processing and hashing and debriefing, set aside some moments when workers can honor what is going well, what they are truly grateful for. Many workplaces have shared with me that they keep morale high by creating systems, formal or informal, that allow workers to praise and thank one another. Such systems could include a bulletin board where people can be anonymously acknowledged, an employee-of-the-week lunch, or simply a culture where people thank each other routinely. Che Guevara, the Argentinean-born Marxist revolutionary, said, "Let me say, at the risk of seeming ridiculous, that the true revolutionary is guided by great feelings of love."

Our acknowledgments to those who help us to be who we are can go such a long way. As the author and AIDS activist Alan Gurganus wrote, "One day on the subway, I stood reading how Reinhold Niebuhr, when asked to define Sainthood, answered, 'The spouses of saints.'" Even as we try to hold it together at work, our personal relationships often begin to suffer—whether they are with friends, partners, children, or other family members. Making an effort to hold our intimate connections in a space of gratitude is an important step.

In our work, too, few things can sustain us as well as gratitude. In Mexico, I met a man who was in large part responsible for the conservation of sea turtles in the Playa San Francisco region. When I asked him if he felt thrilled by what he'd accomplished, he shook his head slowly. "You know, for the first five years I just kept trying to turn it over to someone else in the community so I could leave and go do other things. The next five years I was resigned to staying, but I was resentful and wished someone would come along to take it over. Finally, for the last five years I've accepted being here, and I really appreciate what we get to do day-to-day."

For the purposes of our discussion, we can assume that we've all made a choice to do the work we're doing. It could follow, then, that we may be thankful for the opportunity and that we may experience being able to do the work as an honor. While it may seem like a reach to feel grateful while you fill out random paperwork or negotiate with belligerent public employees, one approach is to ask yourself, "What is the alternative to gratitude?"

Buddhist teachers remind us that there are abundant opportunities for gratitude in even the most mundane aspects of our lives. Thich Nhat Hanh, for example, provides a lesson in washing dishes. As he's scrubbing, he reminds himself that he is grateful for the water, for the opportunity to eat, and for the food he consumed. He goes so far as to say, "Wash each dish as if you are washing the baby Buddha. Why not?"

If we were not raised to see life from this perspective, it can take considerable energy to shift our thinking. And yet if we don't choose to feel honored by our work, the alternative is that we may end up on the road to feeling like someone owes us something, that we're not getting what we're entitled to, or that our work is persecuting us. And that is not a road that goes anywhere we want to go.

It is important, of course, to address the individual and institutional issues connected to our experience. Countless workers do indeed deserve many, many things they are not receiving, including decent wages, benefits, and a healthy work environment. Around the world, there are a multitude of underfunded, underresourced programs doing invisible, undervalued work. Organizations and movements often refuse to say no to taking on more, and then they pass on their overwhelming burden to individual workers and participants. This is where the Buddhist instruction to "wake up to the present moment" is invaluable. We must decide, sometimes multiple times a day, if we can continue to work with the immediate situation as it is, whether or not that situation simultaneously permits us to work for the larger systemic and social change that may one day alter our circumstances. Our integrity and values and ethics cannot be put on hold until we finally get everything we need to do this work. That day may never come.

While we're not so naïve as to believe that injustice and unfairness in either the world or the workplace will instantly disappear, we must ask ourselves, can we bring light and wellness to our work and accomplish the specific tasks that our work requires? Or, in this situation, are they mutually exclusive? For many of us, a persistent feeling of avoidance—as opposed to gratitude—may be a clue that this balance is beyond our reach.

TRY THIS

1. At both the beginning and end of your workday, take a distinct moment to think of one thing you are grateful for.
2. Every single day, think of one person you are grateful to and tell that person so. You can start with those close to you and slowly branch out to expressing your gratitude for all the "teachers" in your life.
3. Advocate for your workplace to create a forum where you and your colleagues can express gratitude to one another. This could be a facilitated time during staff meetings or it could be a bulletin board where employees can post anonymous thank-you notes. Take the lead in thanking others.

CHAPTER TWELVE

THE FIFTH DIRECTION • A Daily Practice of Centering Ourselves

There are only so many ways to commit suicide when you're 13 years old. Or so I thought. I've never been the most creative person, but what I lacked in innovative thinking, I made up for with time. I had so much time to think about how to end my life. It was the only way I could fall asleep at night during what turned out to be the last year of my mom's life. Each night I'd go from *She can't die. She won't die. There's no way she'll die. Please live. Please live. Please live.* to *If she does die, I cannot live. How will I kill myself?* Daily, that was how I centered myself. Every night, that was how I fell asleep. In terms of preventing this catastrophe, it seemed only two things were possible: Either I would find the cure for cancer, or God would appear and intervene. While I would have done anything to cure cancer, my bets were on God appearing. I knew that others died of cancer. But not my mom. She was my whole world. Your whole world can't just end one day, can it?

Three years from when she'd been diagnosed with cancer, and two years and nine months from when they said she'd most likely die, she did die. And my world, as I knew it, ended. Although I did not commit suicide, something bleak and incredibly life altering did happen. I lost all the trust and faith I had. Because the truth was, no matter how sick my mother had gotten, I had clung to my belief that the worst would not happen. I continued to trust. I stayed strong in my faith.

When she died, my trust and faith disappeared and I began to live exclusively in my head. My heart was uninhabitable, so I found refuge in my mind. I was endlessly vigilant. I focused my energy on controlling my surroundings. I managed my new reality by trying to will into existence a way to move through each day. I was entirely uncentered. For anyone who can relate to this, you know that substituting an external architecture for an internal sense of structure can be bulletproof for a time. But only for a time.

Nineteen years later, I would have an opportunity to realize that my faith and trust were not gone entirely, only buried—deep, deep down. Once again I found myself fervently repeating, *Please live. Please live. Please live.* This time I was pleading with my firstborn child, who was being pried from my womb by three sets of doctors' hands. The labor had been 36 hours long. Having had the honor of watching several friends give birth by that point, I knew, intellectually, that anything can happen during labor and delivery. But that didn't count for much in the face of that willful part of my being that had flourished since my mom's death. It kept insisting that, *of all things,* I could deliver a baby on my own. This is perhaps one of women's most ancient beliefs, and for me it was totally unconscious, but it was deeply held nonetheless. The hospital assistance was a nice touch, I thought, but there was no way I was going to be someone who actually needed it.

So on that night, sprawled under impossibly bright lights, numb from my chest down, listening as they cut me open, hearing them agree that "this baby is nowhere near coming out," knowing they were trying to pull my child out of me, I had an epiphany. I could only survive this through faith and trust. *Faith and trust.* Faith and trust—where was I going to find them? For the last 19 years, I'd found all comfort by seeking things outside of myself. By trying to control things. Control and faith don't coexist well, and control was not going to work here. I could not move. Even my tears were being wiped away by someone else—a saintly anesthesiologist. I couldn't micromanage these people; I knew nothing about their craft. I could not think clearly, and what was there to think about? There was only one contribution I could make to this situation, and that was to keep my own heart beating. And so I went deep inside.

I focused on my breathing and going deeper, breathing and going deeper, until I arrived at some unfathomable place that contained what had been locked away for almost two decades: my sense that there was indeed something larger in which I might feel faith and trust. In those moments, which seemed to last an eternity, I remembered what it felt like to be centered. I was humbled; if my life and my baby's life were to be saved, it would be by others, most of whom I didn't know. I felt grateful; their voices sounded as if it would all be okay. I kept breathing. I had not been centered in humility, gratitude, and faith for a long, long time. I had been living in my head, and my heart had been asleep.

While my mother's death and my baby's birth were not experiences that lasted indefinitely, their legacy has. In those moments of becoming a mother, I was brought to my knees, and on some level, I have never gotten up. I can still micromanage and be controlling and live in fear with the best of them, and yet I was able to find a center again, something I thought I had lost with my mom. For me, being centered has come to mean being able to call up that place of humility, gratitude, and trust innumerable times each day. It is what guides any mindfulness I'm able to muster, and it's where I return when I am most challenged.

And this brings us, finally, to the fifth direction. The four directions ultimately lead to the fifth. This direction leads us inside to our core, where we center ourselves, and then, gracefully, leads us back out, renewed in a way that allows us to engage with the outside world at our best. The frequency with which we choose to come home to ourselves and then go out again will vary for everyone. It is my hope that the four directions will aid you in having more and more and more access to the fifth direction—your most awakened self. Many of us are familiar with living in our heads, depending on our intellect, and developing enough external architecture to function and get by. But if we are to truly care for ourselves in a sustainable way, let alone anyone else—if we are to *thrive*—then something greater is required of us. We must discover an awareness of what allows us to live, moment by moment, from a centered place, from an awakened heart.

Throughout history, sages have said that the means to find our truths are already in our possession. We are all capable of creating a daily practice to center ourselves. Eventually, this may allow us to reconnect with the parts of ourselves that feel wise, resourceful, and even divine. A practice may occupy two minutes or two hours, but the hope is that this is something to which you can commit. Your practice will change over time, but what is important is that you prioritize this communion with yourself enough that you come home to yourself daily, if not several times a day.

As almost all of us know, this is easier said than done. Even when we base our practice around something we might find joyful, like singing or riding our bikes, we are likely to resist the commitment. A doctor in a First Nations health services clinic echoed what many of us might say as we describe our attempts to follow through with any piece of a daily practice: "I've done yoga for years. I mean, I haven't done it for a long time. Well, I do it in my head." When challenged as to why he hadn't made it to the gym in months, a community-activist friend of mine said, "I like the *idea* of running." (Figure 12.1)

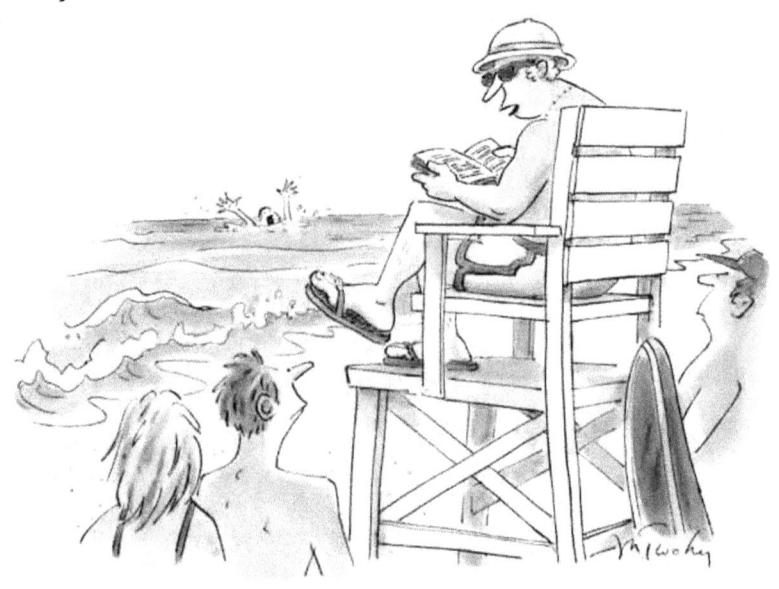

Figure 12.1: "We're encouraging people to become involved in their own rescue"

From my perspective, a practice is not just a healthy option; it is our best hope of creating a truly sustainable life for ourselves. The more often we remind ourselves of this, the more likely we are to discover the discipline we need. Of course, there will be times when our commitment will falter. As our practice deepens, however, we are likely to improve our skills at rebalancing ourselves when we stumble.

As you begin, I would like to suggest two simple techniques that can serve as the first steps toward practice—or even serve as a practice in themselves. The first is to create an intention for your day, and the second is to begin to cultivate moments of mindfulness. Both can be done in a matter of seconds, require no physical exertion, and don't cost a thing. It takes less work to do them than to come up with the excuses to avoid them.

We can stop and create an intention for any aspect of our lives. As a boy, Deepak Chopra watched the practitioners who regularly rose before dawn to gather for daily meditations. In *The Book of Secrets,* he explains that by greeting the sun upon its arrival, the meditators believed they could influence the day. Every morning, they expressed an intention for meeting their purpose that day. For us, too, creating an intention is like allowing sunlight to flood the next few steps in front of us.

We could say: I will notice one thing to find joy in today. I will go to the gym. I will refrain from gossiping. I will move just a little bit slower today. I will smoke fewer cigarettes today than yesterday. A daily intention can focus on a mood or an action. Our goal may be small, but our spirit should be large. We don't know where we will end up, and we certainly don't know how we will get there, but by creating a deliberate intention about what we want for our next hour, next meeting, next interaction, or next day, we are participating in a powerful process of centering ourselves.

In starting with small intentions, we recognize the realities of our lives—how harried or overwhelmed we are, and how difficult it is to remain in the present moment. Even after years of practice, we may still have ways of being that take us far away from where we'd like to be. All my life, for example, I have been impatient. I suppose you could say my impatience feeds the fire that I bring to my life and work, and it has fueled my ability to keep on keeping on at times. But there's been a cost—not only to myself internally, but also in relationships of all kinds in my life. I had my first profound glimpse into the depth of my impatience a few years ago when I had an epiphany about an unconscious belief. I had never imagined myself living past 44, the age my mother was when she died. When I connected the dots, I understood that I didn't expect to be around for a long time, and so I was trying to cram an entire lifetime into a few years. I hurtled through my days and nights at a speed that kept me out of the present moment in fundamental ways.

In recent years, I've found a new set of teachers to educate me about this aspect of my character—my children. As they've grown, no longer able to be directed in the way that was possible when they were younger, the number of times I find myself screaming about this or that has increased exponentially. I'm usually yelling because something is not happening fast enough or in the way I want it to be happening. Instead of coming into the present moment and trying to solve the problem creatively, I let the frustration take over.

One morning recently, I was going off about who knows what. My daughters have grown up immersed in a variety of spiritual practices, but I learned on this day that one in particular had really made an impact on my four-year-old. She's been to multiple meditation retreats, where quite frequently a beautiful bell is rung and everyone stops in their tracks for several minutes at a time. This bell is designed to bring everyone back into the present moment. My daughter has seen thousands of people stop in mid-sentence, mid-movement, mid-step. We'd never talked about this at length, but it apparently took root in her mind.

So there I was, at the height of my diatribe, and suddenly I heard from her mouth a loud "Gonnnngggggg!" She was standing with her feet together, hands folded one on top of the other with her palms up, eyes softly closed, and with the slightest smile across her lips, not unlike a statue of the Buddha. I stopped in mid-yell and began to follow my breath in and out. My shoulders dropped a bit, my heart rate slowed. My seven-year-old relaxed into her breath as well. Minutes passed, and then again we heard my younger daughter sound her definitive "Gonnnngggggg!" We all opened our eyes. Having been returned to the present moment, I found a new direction to take.

This brings us to our second technique. Allowing ourselves to hear the bells that can bring us back to this present moment will greatly influence our ability to practice trauma stewardship. My daughter gave me the gift of functioning as a living "mindfulness bell," but we can also ring those bells for ourselves. Your method can be as seemingly contrived as setting an hourly alarm on your watch, reminding you to stop and pause for a minute; or making a resolution to hear a mental bell that will remind you to choose your words carefully each time you're about to speak; or dividing up your day into thirds so that the beginning, middle, and end are marked by several minutes of "bell time."

The world can be remade to these sounds.

We know that much of the harm in the world is the result of our failure to be present. If we are not present, we cannot achieve the state of integration between our felt sense and our rational mind that will allow us to be deliberate and intentional with our speech, actions, and conduct. Our lack of internal integration often paves the way for decisions, policies, and movements that can create generations of harm.

The possibilities for practice are nearly infinite. Whether we root ourselves in meditation, cooking, prayer, playing the saxophone, lifting weights, or walking our dog, a daily practice can lay the foundation for our work as trauma stewards. Our capacity to help reform our organizations, our communities, our movements, and ourselves is fundamentally altered when we initiate each step from an intentional place within. I think of this as our responsibility. Remembering how high the stakes are with the people we are trying to assist, the creatures we are trying to help, and the planet we are trying to protect, it seems that the *least* we can do is to participate in some kind of a daily (or daily-ish) practice. This is what allows us to bring our best to what we do.

The American Catholic peace activist James Forest said, "What American peace activists might learn from their Vietnamese counterparts is that, until there is a more meditative dimension in the peace movement, our perception of reality (and thus our ability to help occasion understanding and transformation) will be terribly crippled. Whatever our religious or nonreligious background and vocabulary may be, we will be overlooking something as essential to our lives and work as breath itself."

PROFILE HARRY SPENCE

CURRENTLY: Lecturer, Harvard Graduate School of Education and Harvard Kennedy School.

**FORMERLY: Commissioner of the Massachusetts Department of

Social Services; deputy chancellor for operations for the New York City Department of Education; a governor-appointed receiver for the bankrupt city of Chelsea, Massachusetts; a court-appointed receiver for the Boston Housing Authority.

I first started understanding trauma exposure when I began doing child welfare work, which was in December of 2001. I came to the position of commissioner [which he held when we talked] with strikingly little experience in this field, and mostly all I knew about child welfare was from the tabloids. I realized that I was entering this incredibly complex world of utterly imponderable decisions. I was first aware of the quality of decisions that I and the caseworkers were asked to make on a routine basis. I prided myself as a manager on always being able to frame a problem in a way that led to a rationally defined set of solutions, and yet here I was making decisions I couldn't possibly create a rubric for.

I was stunned by how utterly imponderable these decisions are. This is why the story of the wisdom of Solomon is a story about a child welfare problem. Child welfare problems require the wisdom of Solomon.

I was very aware of the weight of these decisions, and I started giving a speech around the parallel process of child welfare. When you're a child welfare worker and the chips are down and you're unlucky and the case goes bad, you'll be fired whether it's your fault or not, so our workers' central experience of the workplace is an experience of betrayal by authority, and we're working with kids who can't trust the adults in their life and have experienced a betrayal by authority. There's a second central parallel process in child welfare, around overwhelm: We try to keep the children safe, but the challenges are so huge and the resources so slim that we're overwhelmed, and we can't take care of the children the way we wish. And then we work with families who are overwhelmed and then say the exact same thing about their parenting.

I started thinking about the parallel process and how the culture of the work reflects the culture of the families we work with and how we assume the same habits and same ways of thinking. I began to think about the other pressures, the pressures of trauma and overwhelm and betrayal.

I started really thinking about what it was like to be engaged in trauma and in creating it at the same time, because when you do removal [of a child from his or her home] you're creating trauma, and while you hope that this trauma is less than the trauma the child's been experiencing, you're still creating trauma. So our workers are both the agents of trauma and the objects of trauma, and I thought, why are we doing this to these poor folks?

I used to give a speech in which I talked about what if I were someone who arrived from outer space, and I said, "How do you protect children?" and someone said, we hire 24-year-olds right out of college, give them a month's training, and then they go observe the most complicated families in our culture, and they then have an obligation to predict the future, and if they're wrong they'll carry blood on their hands and they'll be publicly crucified. And if I heard them explain that this is how they protect children, I'd say you have to be out of your mind.

Atrocities to children are the most disturbing events that occur to us as humans. The culture is so horrified—and we should be so horrified, but we become irrationally obsessed with finding someone to blame, and always the child welfare system is the closest party to blame.

Despite what we know about risk management, there is zero tolerance for a failure, and we think if we spend enough time with the press they'll understand. They won't. This is so primal, it's so deep, that the reporters themselves lose their minds. It's a shared phenomenon, culturally, and the crowd becomes mad in the wake of atrocities.

The child welfare system is fundamentally a traumatized enterprise, and because it is so traumatized, it can't learn. When you're in a state of trauma, you don't learn. It's like we're endlessly in a defensive crouch. I asked myself, "Why is it like this, this system?" Because the objects of this work are so politically weak. They have the least possible claim because they're thought of as "bad parents," and so their ability to demand a better system is zero.

Our folks are suffering horrifically because of trauma exposure. Engagement with families who are traumatized, children who are traumatized, and they themselves are both agents and objects of trauma. They are soaked in trauma. This can't help but have a very, very devastating impact on them as human beings.

The first question I asked is, "Why are we asking them to do this alone?

This is crazy. Why aren't we doing this work in teams?" Then this is how naïve I was: I asked some staff to do a survey of the U.S. in terms of who in the child welfare field nationally is doing this work in teams and how can we learn from them. The answer was zero. I was astounded to find that all 50 states do it the same way we do.

We then had a speaker come from New Orleans, which, even before Hurricane Katrina, was the trauma capital of the nation, and in the course of her talk she said child welfare work is trauma work and you can only do trauma work in teams. I thought to myself, "To hell with it, we're going to go do this." We began an experiment in teaming.

There are many models for this. There is the organizational behavior concept that says the work burden should be shared. I'm an attorney and I know that you don't want one set of eyes making core decisions about facts. That is why we have jury systems, because we know humans see/hear things differently. Also, there is diversity theory, which says several different viewpoints understand things better than one. While it is not formalized throughout the system yet, we have teams in some offices on a pilot basis. I continue to struggle with trauma exposure in the sense of debriefing for our staff. How do you support discussion in regard to debriefing on an ongoing basis? I really want to take care around this issue. Most important is that we do no harm in regard to this, and I know that revisiting trauma without doing essential preparatory work increases the trauma. This is one of the things I've struggled with a lot.

I have an hour with every new class of social workers, and I talk about the most important decision they're going to make: It's the decision around what you are going to do with the pain in the work. Generally, there are two ways to address the pain in this work.

One is to simply say I have to learn to be less emotionally vulnerable: If I keep being dragged around by my emotions like by a team of horses, then I need to armor my heart. The problem with this is we work with kids and kids have a preternatural capacity to read your natural state, because their survival depends on their intuitively reading the emotional state of the adults in their lives. If you're emotionally shut down, they'll know it—the vibe will be different. If you're going to work with a child whose experience of adults is that they're unpredictable, dangerous, and disconnected, and if you're removed emotionally, they'll experience you as confirming their worst fears. But it's not only the children who'll be damaged—you'll do damage to yourself. You're going to lose a parent or break up with a partner, and these habits will spill over to your personal life and they don't work.

What's the alternative? I talk a lot about the second way to respond to the pain of this work, and that is by encouraging resiliency and the ability to get back on your feet. I also talk about the work of Bill Beardsley. He says there are three steps to resiliency: self-reflection, relationships, and action. You know you're going to feel overwhelmed in this work and in life, especially nowadays—the question is, what do you do with it, and can you recover from it or do you go into an ongoing state of overwhelm?

When I talk about resiliency, I share this story of going to give a keynote talk, and it was right after a child whom we were involved with had died. I was really disconnected from my body and felt incredibly weird during the talk, and I just couldn't shake this feeling. I was really off. Afterwards, I sat down and wondered what was the matter with me. Once I was still for a few minutes, I felt this huge grief come up inside of me, and I felt intensely sad. I turned to my friend who I was sitting with, and I told him how I was feeling and how I'd been so confused and so upset about this case. This was a good friend, and he said some comforting things to me, and we sat there together. Part of what is important about relationships is that although the grief and pain that has filled the entire screen of my consciousness doesn't disappear, it does become manageable. I can remember that there is support and caring in the world as evidenced through my friend. The bad feelings do not disappear, but they are pulled back to their appropriate proportion, and I can see that while this is definitely part of a picture of my life, the tendency I have for my feelings to overwhelm me is reduced.

I can come back to myself by taking these three steps of self-reflection, being in relationship, and action. Through these steps, then, I remind myself that I'm okay. I'm fine, in fact. I'm just a sad person who is feeling pain. It's not about how to kill the sadness, but to size my feelings so I can manage them and come through them and experience all the other things in life as well as these intense feelings of pain.

We need to know this to help our child welfare families understand this. The ability to model resiliency is crucial. It's what we need to do for ourselves and for our child welfare families. We also need to be able to ask ourselves, "What is the trauma that I witness hooking in me?" Every child has the experience or that emotion of abuse or neglect. Every child has the experience of a caregiver yelling at us unfairly or being really distracted and we feel abused or neglected, so we all know the emotion of abuse and neglect. We need to be aware of how the trauma hooks into our own experience. This needs to be explicitly addressed. I want those who have this experience to be okay with that and be aware of it, because otherwise it'll hook you and drag you around and you won't know what's going on. If you have some awareness, then at least you can understand what's happening by the emotion that comes out of your vicarious experience. We need to continuously be asking ourselves,

"What in this pain is connecting to what in me, and where is that original pain coming from?" We all know that those of us who do this work disproportionately do this work because we've experienced this ourselves.

First thing, you have to be aware of what your emotion even is. It's like with the story I told earlier: Until I let myself feel this experience of grief, I'm just a very distraught human being. The first step in managing the pain is acknowledging it. Then we can connect with others and take action.

It's important to acknowledge that it's not as though organizations that have been deeply traumatized always want to come out from under this trauma. To heal, you have to come out of it, but sometimes they want to stay in it, and they can be very ambivalent about changing. In our situation we have both sides of this ambivalence. We have workers who think, "We do God's work and no one will understand, but that's okay because God will, so I'll just stay isolated." For me, that's where I get my secondary trauma: from that defensive crouch and the isolated worker. It's like that parable of the frog at the bottom of the deep dry well where it is slimy and disgusting and dark and filled with scorpions and snakes, and the frog has learned to jump from rock to rock and live in fear and survive it all. One day he looks up, and in the sunshine at the top of the well is another frog, who looks down and says, "Hey, you should come up here. It's beautiful up here. We've got a lily pond, we can catch flies, and we eat all day—it's blissful up here." The frog at the bottom of the well says, "F---you, that's not reality." In our efforts, we've had both wonderful acceptance and deep ambivalence and real resistance. That's a fairly startling discovery for me.

We have this addiction to all the things we've become habituated to, even though we live in this untenable situation ... same as the families we work with. It's more disturbing for me to see it in staff, because for them it's not very far from the bottom of the well up to the lily pad, but it's because they're so habituated to their circumstances. Also, we in child welfare carry this "rescuing the child from the family" fantasy, which is so horrific and so deep in the culture. The world has no idea what it bit off to chew when it decided to take up child welfare. It's the most complex work that we do, certainly that we do in state government, and the public has no comprehension of it.

Every organization I've ever worked with in my life has been troubled. If you asked the workers, "How serious about this task are you?" if you're lucky, 75 percent of your workforce would say they were serious. In child welfare, it's 99 percent of your workforce. We have huge debates, people are damaged by it, but nobody says, "I'm just sick of this task. I could not care less." The commitment to the task is very intense, and there is very little cynicism about the task.

I am enormously supported in my work by my own spiritual practice. Also, my wife is an organizational behaviorist, and she introduced me to various forms of group dynamics work, including the Tavistock Institute and A.K. Rice's work, which studies and reflects on the covert emotional life of organizations, particularly in relation to authority. The work they do is deeply connected to issues of spiritual practice for me, because much of this is around ego and other quasi-mystical notions. Bessel van der Kolk worked with Bishop Tutu in South Africa, and he says there are a variety of ways that humans manage trauma, and in most of the world it's through bodily movement, often dancing or other things music related. One small portion of the world where trauma is not dealt with that way is Northwest Europe. The tradition there is alcohol. Van der Kolk talked about when he'd attend the Truth and Reconciliation Commission and they'd open up the hearing in the mornings, and it'd start with Tutu singing and then everybody singing, and then they'd dance and after a period then they'd stop, hear a few witnesses sharing unbearable stories, and then Tutu would sing again and dance and then take a few witnesses so that at each step they were managing until they couldn't bear it or hold it any longer, and then they'd sing again and do some sort of bodily movement.

We've begun using Circles in our work. We talk about how explicit to make the spiritual dimension at the beginning of the Circle, but we have a Circle keeper and we talk about creating a sacred space and each person can decide what that means for them. We have sometimes substituted staff meetings with Circles, and we have used Circles with our families as well. We've used them when we've done race work in an effort to support people in feeling safe and to have an ability to speak from the heart. We have a few offices that have been trained in Circles based on First Nation practices, and we've been trained by this phenomenal organization in Boston that does youth development work called Roca.

As far as how I take care of myself, I find it quite fascinating that this work, in a way that no other work I've done has been, is a constant test of how centered I am. If I'm not centered, I am jarred immediately. The work itself becomes a kind of gauge of my spiritual or psychological state. I don't really care whether you think of these issues as spiritual issues or psychological issues. I'm interested in trying to develop an organization in which the concept of spiritual growth or psychological growth is understood to be essential to the leadership of an organization. There is no question that you need to be engaged in self-reflection and growth. How can I develop a public organization that explicitly holds that as a value in leadership?

This work keeps me in touch constantly with where I am spiritually or psychologically. Whichever way I understand it, it keeps me in constant touch with when I'm out of kilter or not centered. When I'm not able to be myself in an authentic way, I feel a jarring sense in the organization, and that pushes me to a spiritual practice or psychological practice that gets me re-centered. Ultimately they're inextricably related. Also I am involved with Learning as Leadership in California, which provides leadership seminars within an immensely powerful individual psychological framework. So this combines with the very powerful group framework that derives from the Tavistock workshops I have done, and also combines with my own spiritual framework. I move among all of these.

If I did not have my spiritual practice, I'd be crazy. Either the way the world thinks of crazy, or the way that most people in power are crazy. My wife does not have a spiritual practice, but we have found ourselves in the same territory even though the language we use is very different. For both of us there is something about deep learning, whether spiritual practice or whatever you call it, that seems to be essential to keeping ourselves able to do what our best selves aspire to do. That relationship with my wife has been crucial. We have a sense of a common task, a sense of a shared task.

Additionally I have a rule that my family takes a month every summer to go to an island in Greece and disappear. I also believe that part of my responsibility is to continuously survey the world in all its various dimensions. If I only do this work all the time, I will greatly limit my capacity to lead the organization and have a larger vision. I am also a deep believer in letting yourself stop thinking about stuff. Take yourself and your mind to a completely different place, and in that process your creativity for bringing solutions to child welfare will increase.

I'm busy. I make myself too busy, I overtask, but not around work. I don't have a television, and that's really important to me. Some of that is about not having internal and external chatter all the time. I also

> have an 11-year-old and we have a pretty quiet home. We take our time with things, and I cook a lot because I find that a wonderfully healing and helpful activity. I have an irregular meditation practice, and I do yoga regularly. I consciously resist being a workaholic.

TRY THIS

1. When your day begins, close your eyes, take several deep breaths, and ask yourself, "What is my intention today?" If you have small children or loud chickens demanding your attention before you are conscious, ask yourself this while feeding your children or gathering the day's eggs, but create an intention for the day.
2. At the end of your day, before sleep overtakes you, ask yourself, "What can I put down? What am I ready to be done with? What don't I need to carry with me for another day?" Put it down, and don't pick it up again the next day.

3. Designate a day of rest. Whether you identify it as Shabbat or the Sabbath or simply a day off, designate a weekly day of non-obligation for yourself. This will serve to remind us that if we are truly to reconnect with ourselves, work and creation must stop. Our day of rest will also remind us that who we are as individuals and as members of society is about our deepest essence and not about what we produce during the week. In addition to your day of rest, allot some time for yourself each day when you don't obligate yourself to anything, but instead give yourself total freedom to delight in one of your favorite states of being. Be present with this for however long you are able. Notice how you feel when you free yourself from obligation and allow yourself to be centered within.

CONCLUSION
Closing Intention

> Don't ask yourself what the world needs. Ask yourself what makes you come alive. And go do that. Because the world needs people who've come alive.
> Howard Thurman, American theologian and civil rights leader

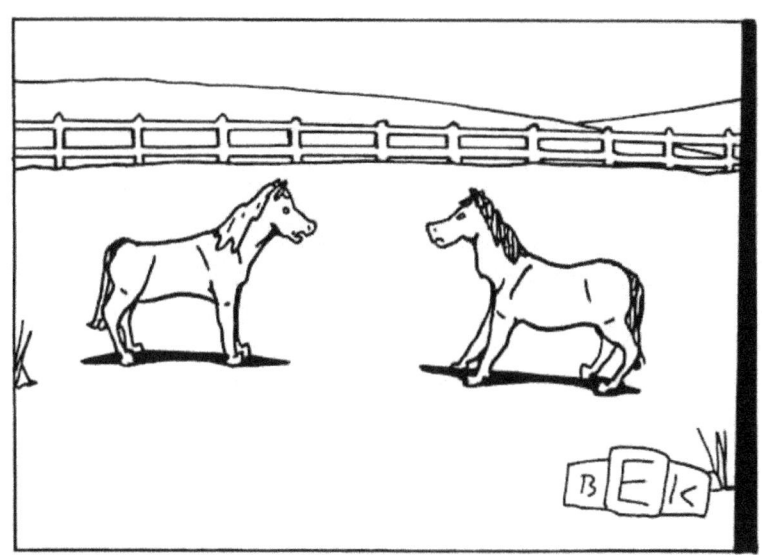

Figure I

At certain times of year in the Pacific Northwest, there are so many spider webs outside in the early morning that it's hard to move without colliding with one of these glorious creations. I try to take my moments of sudden stopping as a reminder of Chief Sealth's insight that we are all a part of a much larger web of life. As we prepare to depart on our separate yet connected journeys of trauma stewardship, it helps to remember that this web of life, as it extends throughout the world, is vast, intricate, and complicated in ways we may not understand.

Because the web of life is too complex for any human being to know completely, people often lose sight of the fact that there is a whole. But there is. And when we look at the spider's creation, it is clear that even the slenderest strand makes a difference to the strength and sustainability of the entire miraculous structure. The same is true for each and every one of us. It *matters* that we try to do no harm. It *matters* that we try to keep our energy moving and healthy. It *matters* that we appreciate life's strength and delicacy. It *matters* that we awaken to the web's presence and then interact with it in an intentional and deliberate way. Otherwise, we will walk right through our own web without ever seeing its beauty, the way it reflects the sunlight or collects the morning dew.

John Muir, a Scottish-born American naturalist, once wrote, "When we try to pick out anything by itself, we find that it is bound fast, by a thousand invisible cords that cannot be broken, to everything else in the Universe."

By now, we know that if we want to decrease the suffering in our world, we will need to learn a behavior that is fundamentally different from the ones that have caused such pain and destruction. We must open ourselves to the suffering that comes with knowing that there are species we can't bring back from extinction, children we can't free from their abusive homes, climate changes we can't reverse, and wounded veterans we can't immediately heal. We must also open ourselves to the hope that comes with understanding the one thing we can do. We can always be present for our lives, the lives of all other beings, and the life of the planet. Being present is a radical act. It allows us to soften the impact of trauma, interrupt the forces of oppression, and set the stage for healing and transformation. Best of all, our quality of presence is something we can cultivate, moment by moment. It permits us to greet what arises in our lives with our most enlightened selves, thereby allowing us to have the best chance of truly repairing the world.

As we continue on our journeys, may our lives be informed by our deepening awareness of our role in life's web. May we care well for ourselves and for others. May we remember that our courage on this path lies in the way we take each and every step. "If one is to do good, it must be done in the minute particulars," said the English poet and artist William Blake. May we remember that trauma stewardship requires us to honor others and our planet in a way that is possible only if we have made a commitment to our own path of wellness. May we discover peace amid the strife, joy amid the suffering, and trust amid the groundlessness that is, ultimately, life's course.

NOTES

Every attempt has been made to accurately cite all of our sources. Trauma Stewardship is based on 20 years of work in the field, both in the United States and abroad, and as there was never a historical intention to write a book, detailed accounts of person, time, and place were not consistently recorded. We have tried to gather as much detail on those sources as is available to us. The author regrets any omissions. During the writing of this edition, several individuals were interviewed who asked to remain anonymous. We have honored their requests.

Langston Hughes poem: Langston Hughes, *The Dream Keeper* (New York: Alfred A. Knopf, 1932).

INTRODUCTION

Seung Sahn: Pipe ceremony experienced by the author, Washington, 2006.

Newsweek article: Eve Conant with Sarah Childress, "To Share in the

Horror," *Newsweek,* March 19, 2007, 34.

CNN.com article: Andree LeRoy, M.D., "Exhaustion, anger of caregiving get a name," CNN.com/health,http://www.cnn.com/2007/HEALTH/conditions/08/13/caregiver.syndrome/index.html(accessed 2007).

Figley: Charles Figley, *Compassion Fatigue: Coping with Secondary Traumatic Stress Disorder in Those Who Treat the Traumatized* (London: Brunner-Routledge, 1995).

Pearlman: Laurie Anne Pearlman, Karen W. Saakvitne, *Trauma and the Therapist: Countertransference and Vicarious Traumatization in Psychotherapy with Incest Survivors* (New York: W.W. Norton & Co, 1995).

Conte: Jon R. Conte, interview by the author, Seattle, WA, 2006.

Dictionary: Merriam-Webster OnLine, http://www.merriam-webster.com/dictionary/stewardship (accessed December 2008).

Journal article: Richard Worrell and Michael Appleby, "Stewardship of Natural Resources: Definition, Ethical and Practical Aspects," *Journal of Agricultural* and *Environmental Ethics* 12, no.3 (2000), http://www.springerlink.com/content/q6x165h4j2276306 (accessed 2006).

E.B. White: E.B. White, *Essays of E.B. White* (NewYork: Harper & Row, 1977).

CHAPTER ONE

Emerson: Ralph Waldo Emerson, *The Complete Works of Ralph Waldo Emerson* (Boston & New York: Houghton Mifflin, 1903–1904).

Kabat-Zinn: Jon Kabat-Zinn, *Wherever You Go, There You Are: Mindfulness Meditation in Everyday Life* (New York: Hyperion, 1994).

Siegel: Daniel J. Siegel, *The Mindful Brain: Reflection and Attunement in the Cultivation of Well-Being.* (New York: W.W. Norton & Co, 2007).

Suzuki Roshi: Jack Kornfield, dharma talk at Spirit Rock Meditation Center, Woodacre, CA, 2002.

Anne Frank: Jack Canfield, Mark Victor Hansen, Nancy Mitchell Autio, LeAnn Thieman, LPN, *Chicken Soup for the Nurse's Soul: 101 Stories to*

Celebrate, Honor, and Inspire the Nursing Profession (New York: HCI, 2001).

Stevie Wonder: Stevie Wonder, in concert, Seattle, WA, July 11, 2008.

CHAPTER TWO

Gandalf quotation: J.R.R. Tolkien, *The Lord of the Rings: The Return of the King* (New York: Houghton Mifflin, 1999).

Golie Jansen: Golie Jansen, "Vicarious Trauma and Its Impact on Advocates, Therapists, and Friends," *Research & Advocacy* Digest 6, no.2 (2004).

Michael Lipsky: Michael Lipsky, *Street-Level Bureaucracy: Dilemmas of the Individual in Public Services* (New York: Russell Sage Foundation, 1983).

Street-level bureaucrat: Lipsky, *Street-Level Bureaucracy.*

Beth Richie: Beth E. Richie, Ph.D, interview by the author, Seattle, WA, 2006.

The *New York Times Magazine:* Benjamin Weiser, "The Wrong Man,"

New York Times Magazine, August 6, 2000: 30–35, 48, 60–63.

Flateau and Gangi: Benjamin Weiser, "State to Pay in Case of Man Wrongly Held," *New York Times,* http://query.nytimes.com/gst/fullpage.html?res=9803E0DB1231 F930A25757C0A9679C8B63&sec=&spon= (accessed April 13, 2001).

Structural violence: Johan Galtung, "Violence, Peace, and Peace Research," *Journal of Peace Research* 6.3 (1969): 167–91.

Paul Farmer: Paul Farmer, *Pathologies of Power: Health, Human Rights, and the New War on the Poor* (Berkeley: University of California Press, 2004).

Caregiver stress: Andree LeRoy, M.D., "Exhaustion, anger of caregiving get a name," CNN.com/health, http://www.cnn.com/2007/HEALTH/conditions/08/13/caregiver.syndrome/index.html (accessed 2007).

McFarlane and van der Kolk: Bessel A. van der Kolk, Alexander C. McFarlane, and Lars Weisaeth, eds., *Traumatic Stress: The Effects of Overwhelming Experience on Mind,*

Body, and Society (New York: Guilford Press, 1996).
Trauma and its challenge to society: Van der Kolk, McFarlane, and Weisaeth, *Traumatic Stress.*

CHAPTER THREE

Mo O'Brien: Mo O'Brien, interview by the author, New Orleans, LA, 2006.

Laurie Leitch: Laurie Leitch, Ph.D., interview by the author, Seattle, WA, 2006.

Brian Bride: University of Georgia, "Social Workers May Indirectly Experience Post-traumatic Stress," *ScienceDaily,* January 10, 2007, http://www.science daily.com/releases/2007/0 1/070104144711.htm (accessed 2007).

Ray Suarez interview: Archbishop Desmond Tutu, interview by Ray Suarez, *Talk of the Nation,* National Public Radio, November 23, 1998.

Waking the Tiger: Peter Levine, *Waking the Tiger—Healing Trauma* (Berkeley: North Atlantic Books, 1997).

Branford Marsalis: Branford Marsalis, interview for film documentary *Jazz,* produced by Ken Burns and Lynn Novick and written by Geoffrey Ward (Florentine Films and WETA, Washington, D.C., in association with BBC, 2000).

CHAPTER FOUR

Karen Lips: Karen Lips, personal communication, October 2008.

Victor Pantesco: Victor Pantesco, personal communication, 2008.

Kirsten Stade: Kirsten Stade, interview by the author, Seattle, WA, October, 2008.

Garber and Seligman: Judy Garber and Martin E.P. Seligman, *Human Helplessness: Theory and Applications* (San Diego, CA: Academic Press, 1980).

Subway ads: New York City Administration for Children's Services, with kind permission, May 8, 2008.

Luo Lan: Luo Lan, personal communication, October 2008.

Elaine Miller-Karas: Elaine Miller-Karas, interview by the author, Seattle, WA, 2006.

Stephanie Levine: Stephanie Levine, personal communication, 2006.

Alice and the Queen: Lewis Carroll, *Alice's Adventures in Wonderland and Through the Looking-Glass* (New York: Penguin Classics, 2003).

X-Files: David Duchovny and Chris Carter, "The Sixth Extinction II: Amor Fati [Love of Fate]," *The X-Files*, aired November 14, 1999.

Billie Lawson: Billie Lawson, interview by the author, Seattle, WA, 2000.

Learned to make my mind large: Maxine Hong Kingston, *The Woman Warrior* (New York: Vintage Books, 1976).

Thich Nhat Hanh: "Nomination of Thich Nhat Hanh for Nobel Peace Prize," Martin Luther King Jr., January 25, 1967, http://www.hartford-hwp.com/archives/45a/025.html (accessed 2006).

Letter from Thich Nhat Hanh: Plum Village Monastery, France, August 8, 2006, with kind permission.

Kati Loeffler: Kati Loeffler, personal communication, 2008.

Trauma Center in Boston: The Trauma Center Resources, "Police Stress," Trauma Center at Justice Resource Institute, http://www.traumac

enter.org/resources/pdf_files/Police_Stress.pdf (accessed 2006).

R. Omar Casimire: R. Omar Casimire, interview by the author, post-Katrina, 2005.

Newsweek article: Eve Conant with Sarah Childress, "To Share in the Horror," *Newsweek,* March 19, 2007, 34.

Holocaust survivor: Rabbi, personal communication, 2002.

Diane Tatum: Diane Tatum, personal communication, 1999.

Thich Nhat Hanh dharma talk: Thich Nhat Hanh, *Being Peace* (Berkeley: Parallax Press, 2002).

Hafiz: Hafiz, *The Gift,* Daniel Ladinsky, trans. (New York: Penguin, 1999).

Dune: *Dune,* written and directed by David Lynch, from the novel by Frank Herbert (Universal Studios, 1984).

Star Wars: Star Wars: Episode I—The Phantom Menace, written and directed by George Lucas (Lucasfilm, 1999), http://www.imdb.com/title/tt0120915/quotes (accessed November 18, 2008).

John Petersen: From teacher, personal communication, 2004.

When you see the suffering: From teacher, personal communication, 2002.

Jon Conte: Jon Conte, interview by the author, Seattle, WA, 2000.

Thomas Merton: Thomas Merton, *Conjectures of a Guilty Bystander* (New York: Image, Doubleday, 1968).

Shantideva: Pema Chödrön, dharma talk, Berkeley, CA, 2002.

Ginny NiCarthy: Ginny NiCarthy, personal communication, 2006.

Karyn Schwartz: Karyn Schwartz, personal communication, 2006.

CHAPTER FIVE

Chance has never yet: Amy Jacques-Garvey, ed., "Philosophy and Opinions of Marcus Garvey," 1923, http://www.Wordowner.com/garvey (accessed November 18, 2008).

Pema Chödrön: Pema Chödrön, *The Places That Scare You* (Boston: Shambhala Publications, 2001).

Peter Levine: Peter Levine, *Waking the Tiger—Healing Trauma,* (Berkeley: North Atlantic Books, 1997).

Jack Kornfield: Jack Kornfield, dharma talk, Spirit Rock Meditation Center, Woodacre, CA, 2002.

Stress-resistant persons: Bessel A. van der Kolk, *Psychological Trauma* (Arlington, VA: American Psychiatric Press, 1987).

Martin Luther King Jr.: Martin Luther King Jr., Washington State University, Dr. Martin Luther King Jr. Community Celebration, http://mlk.Wsu.edu/default.Asp?PageID=1481 (accessed November 19, 2008).

CHAPTER SIX

Abandon any hope of fruition: Pema Chödrön, dharma talk, Berkeley, CA, 2002.

Peter Levine: Peter Levine, *Waking the Tiger—Healing Trauma,* (Berkeley: North Atlantic Books, 1997).

Integrated state: Daniel J. Siegel, interview by the author, Seattle, WA, 2008.

Charles Newcomb: Charles Newcomb, personal communication.

Dr. Liu Dong: Dr. Liu Dong, qigong retreat, Seattle, WA, 2006.

Kenneth Cohen: Kenneth Cohen, *The Way of Qigong: The Art and Science of Chinese Energy Healing* (New York: Ballantine Books, 1999).

Dr. Liu Dong: Dr. Liu Dong, qigong retreat, Seattle, WA, 2006.

CHAPTER EIGHT

Nietzsche: Viktor Frankl, *Man's Search for Meaning* (Boston: Beacon Press, 1959).

Could this be why: John Brookins, personal communication, 2007.

Although firsthand experience: Bessel A. van der Kolk, Alexander C. McFarlane, and Lars Weisaeth, eds., *Traumatic Stress: The Effects of Overwhelming Experience on Mind, Body, and Society* (New York: Guilford Press, 1996).

With love to my: Peter van Dernoot, *Helping Your Children Cope with Your Cancer: A Guide for Parents and Families* (Long Island City: Hatherleigh Press, 2002).

James Mooney: James Mooney, personal communication, 1999.

Al Gore: Al Gore, *An Inconvenient Truth* (Paramount Classics, 2006).

Zaid Hassan: Zaid Hassan, personal communication, 2006.

John Brookins: John Brookins, personal communication, 2007.

Viktor Frankl: Viktor Frankl, *Man's Search for Meaning* (Boston: Beacon Press, 1959).

CHAPTER NINE

The real voyage: Marcel Proust, *Remembrance of Things Past: Three Book Boxed Set—The Definitive French Pleiade Edition,* C.K. Moncrieff, Terence Kilmartin, Andreas Mayor, trans. (New York: Vintage Books/Random House, 1982).

Deepak Chopra: Deepak Chopra, The Book of Secrets: Unlocking the Hidden Dimensions of Your Life (New York: Harmony Books, 2004).

Rubin "Hurricane" Carter: From *The Hurricane* (Universal Pictures, 1999).

Mark Lilly: Mark Lilly, interview by the author, Seattle, WA, 2008.

William James: William James, *The Principles of Psychology,* Volume 1 (New York: Cosimo Classics, 2007).

Viktor Frankl: Viktor Frankl, *Man's Search for Meaning* (Boston: Beacon Press, 1959).

Rumi: Jan Phillips, *Divining the Body: Reclaim the Holiness of Your Physical Self* (Woodstock, VT: SkyLight Paths Publishing, 2005).

Plan B Skateboards: Mike Ternasky, interview by the author, Seattle, WA, 2006.

CHAPTER TEN

Peter Senge: Peter M. Senge, *The Dance of Change: The Challenges to Sustaining Momentum in Learning Organizations* (New York: Doubleday, 1999).

Traumatic Stress: Bessel A. van der Kolk, Alexander C. McFarlane, and Lars Weisaeth, eds., *Traumatic Stress: The Effects of Overwhelming Experience on Mind, Body, and Society* (New York: Guilford Press, 1996).

I, for one, believe: Malcolm X, February 14, 1965, from Patricia

Robinson, "Malcolm X, Our Revolutionary Son and Brother," in *Malcolm X: The Man and His Times,* ed. John Henrik Clarke (New York: Macmillan, 1969), 56–63 (Trenton, NJ: Africa World Press, 1990).

If your compassion: Jack Kornfield, dharma talk at Spirit Rock Meditation Center, Woodacre, CA, 2002.

Chief Sealth: Chief Sealth, speech to a representative of the U.S. government, 1854.

Archbishop Desmond Tutu: Archbishop Desmond Tutu, interview by Ray Suarez, *Talk of the Nation,* National Public Radio, November 23, 1998.

Jill Robinson: Jill Robinson, interview by the author, Seattle, WA, October 2008.

Kufunda: Marianne Knuth, interview by the author, Seattle, WA, 2006; Kufunda Learning Village, http://www.kufunda.org/whatandwhy.php?sheet=1 (accessed 2006).

Architecture for Humanity: Cameron Sinclair and Kate Stohr, interview by the author, Seattle, WA, 2006; Architecture for Humanity, http://www.

Architectureforhumanity.org/about (accessed 2006).

CHAPTER ELEVEN

Leonardo da Vinci: Michael J. Gelb, *How to Think Like Leonardo da Vinci: Seven Steps to Genius Every Day* (New York: Dell Publishing, 2000).

The Daily Tao: Deng Ming-Dao, 365 Tao—Daily Meditations, http://www.fortunecity.com/roswell/vortex/401/library/365/365date.htm (accessed 2005).

Peter Levine: Peter Levine, *Waking the Tiger—Healing Trauma* (Berkeley: North Atlantic Books, 1997).

Jack Kornfield: Jack Kornfield, dharma talk at Spirit Rock Meditation Center, Woodacre, CA, 2002.

Thich Nhat Hanh: Thich Nhat Hanh, dharma talk at Deer Park Monastery, Escondido, CA, 2004.

The ordinary response to atrocities: Judith Herman, *Trauma and Recovery: The Aftermath of Violence—from Domestic Abuse to Political Terror* (New York: Basic Books, 1997).

Richards and Taylor-Murphy: Kimberley Richards and Kanika

Taylor-Murphy, personal communication, 2006.

Clifton Fadiman: Terry L. Paulson, *Making Humor Work: Take Your Job Seriously and Yourself Lightly* (Los Altos, CA: Crisp Publications, 1995).

Steven Sultanoff: Steven Sultanoff, personal communication, January 3, 2009.

Leo Rosten: Ilan Stavans, "O Rosten! My Rosten!" *Pakn Treger* 52 (Fall 2006), National Yiddish Book Center, http://www.yiddishbookcenter.org/pdf/pt/52/PT52_rosten.pdf.

James Thurber: Max Eastman, *Enjoyment of Laughter* (New York: Simon and Schuster, 1936).

Margie Brown: Terry L. Paulson, *Making Humor Work: Take Your Job Seriously and Yourself Lightly* (Los Altos, CA: Crisp Publications, 1995).

Che Guevara: Shane Claiborne, *The Irresistible Revolution: Living as an Ordinary Radical* (Grand Rapids, MI: Zondervan, 2006).

Alan Gurganus: Alan Gurganus, *Plays Well with Others* (New York: Random House, 1997).

Thich Nhat Hanh: Thich Nhat Hanh, dharma talk at Deer Park Monastery, Escondido, CA, 2004.

CHAPTER TWELVE

Deepak Chopra: Deepak Chopra, *The Book of Secrets: Unlocking the Hidden Dimensions of Your Life* (New York: Harmony Books, 2004).

James Forest: William H. Houff, *Infinity in Your Hand* (Boston: Unitarian Universalist Association of Congregations, 1994).

CONCLUSION

Howard Thurman: "An Invitation, Not a Threat," sermon preached by the Rev. William McD. Tully, rector, St. Bartholomew's Church, New York, December 2, 2007, http://stbarts.org/images/Sermons_Text/ser120207_11am.pdf (accessed January 4, 2009).

John Muir: Sierra Club, "The Life and Contributions of John Muir," http://www.sierraclub.org/john_muir_exhibit/ (accessed October 2008).

William Blake: Jack Kornfield, The Art of Forgiveness, Lovingkindness, and Peace (New York: Bantam Books, 2002).

SELECTED BIBLIOGRAPHY

This is a list of books that readers may find especially useful as they explore the issues related to trauma stewardship. It contains most of the major works referred to in the text, as well as supplemental sources that readers may find helpful. And, of course, this book has been informed by other sources, unfortunately too numerous to list here.

Cameron, Anne. *Daughters of Copper Woman.* Vancouver, British Columbia: Press Gang Publishing, 1981.

Canfield, Jack, Mark Victor Hansen, Nancy Mitchell Autio, LeAnn Thieman, LPN. *Chicken Soup for the Nurse's Soul: 101 Stories to Celebrate, Honor, and Inspire the Nursing Profession.* New York: HCI, 2001.

Chödrön, Pema. *The Places That Scare You.* Boston: Shambhala Publications, 2001.

———. *When Things Fall Apart.* New York: Shambhala, 1997.

Chopra, Deepak. *The Book of Secrets: Unlocking the Hidden Dimensions of Your Life.* New York: Harmony Books, 2004.

Cohen, Kenneth S. *The Way of Qigong: The Art and Science of Chinese Energy Healing.* New York: Ballantine Books, 1999.

Dalai Lama. *The Compassionate Life.* Somerville, MA: Wisdom Publications, 2001.

Emerson, Ralph Waldo. *The Complete Works of Ralph Waldo Emerson.* Boston & New York: Houghton Mifflin, 1903–1904.

Farmer, Paul. *Pathologies of Power: Health, Human Rights, and the New War on the Poor.* Berkeley: University of California Press, 2004.

Figley, Charles R. *Compassion Fatigue: Coping with Secondary Traumatic Stress*

Disorder in Those Who Treat the Traumatized. London: Brunner-Routledge, 1995.

Frankl, Viktor. *Man's Search for Meaning.* Boston: Beacon Press, 1959.

Gandhi, Mohandas K., Mahadev Desai, trans. *Autobiography: The Story of My Experiments with Truth.* Boston: Beacon Press, 1983.

Garber, Judy, and Martin E.P. Seligman. *Human Helplessness: Theory and Applications.* San Diego: Academic Press, 1980.

Herman, Judith. *Trauma and Recovery: The Aftermath of Violence—from Domestic Abuse to Political Terror.* New York: Basic Books, 1997.

Hughes, Langston. *The Dream Keeper.* New York: Alfred A. Knopf, 1932.

Garber, Judy, and Martin E.P. Seligman. *Human Helplessness: Theory and Applications.* San Diego, CA: Academic Press, 1980.

Gurganus, Alan. *Plays Well with Others.* New York: Random House, 1997.

James, William. *The Principles of Psychology, Volume 1.* New York: Cosimo Classics, 2007.

Kabat-Zinn, Jon. *Wherever You Go, There You Are: Mindfulness Meditation in Everyday Life.* New York: Hyperion, 1994.

Kahn, William A. *Holding Fast: The Struggle to Create Resilient Caregiving Organizations.* New York: Brunner-Routledge, 2005.

Kingston, Maxine Hong. *The Woman Warrior.* New York: Vintage Books, 1976.

Kornfield, Jack. *A Path with Heart: A Guide Through the Perils and Promises of Spiritual Life.* New York: Bantam Books, 1993.

Levine, Peter. *Waking the Tiger—Healing Trauma.* Berkeley: North Atlantic Books, 1997.

Lipsky, Michael. *Street-Level Bureaucracy: Dilemmas of the Individual in Public Services.* New York: Russell Sage Foundation, 1983.

Maathai, Wangari. *Unbowed.* New York: Random House, 2006.

Mandela, Nelson. *Long Walk to Freedom: The Autobiography of Nelson Mandela.* Boston: Little, Brown and Company, 1995.

Merton, Thomas. *Conjectures of a Guilty Bystander.* New York: Image, Doubleday, 1968.

Moraga, Cherríe, and Gloria Anzaldúa. *This Bridge Called My Back: Writings by Radical Women of Color.* Pittsburgh: Persephone Press, 1981.

NiCarthy, Ginny. *Getting Free—You Can End Abuse and Take Back Your Life.* Emeryville, CA: Seal Press, 1982.

Pearlman, Laurie Anne, and Karen W. Saakvitne. *Trauma and the Therapist: Countertransference and Vicarious*

Traumatization in Psychotherapy with Incest Survivors. New York: W.W. Norton & Co, 1995.

Richie, Beth E. *Compelled to Crime: The Gender Entrapment of Battered Black Women.* New York: Routledge, 1996.

Senge, Peter M. *The Dance of Change: The Challenges to Sustaining Momentum in Learning Organizations.* New York: Doubleday, 1999.

Siegel, Daniel J. *The Mindful Brain: Reflection and Attunement in the Cultivation of Well-Being.* New York: W.W. Norton & Co, 2007.

Sinclair, Cameron, and Kate Stohr. *Design Like You Give a Damn: Architectural Responses to Humanitarian Crises.* New York: Metropolis Books, 2006.

Thich Nhat Hanh. *Being Peace.* Berkeley: Parallax Press, 2002.

_____. *The Miracle of Mindfulness.* Boston: Beacon Press, 1999.

Tolkien, J.R.R. *The Lord of the Rings: The Return of the King.* New York: Houghton Mifflin, 1999.

Tutu, Desmond. *No Future Without Forgiveness.* New York: Doubleday, 1999.

van der Kolk, Bessel A. *Psychological Trauma.* Arlington, VA: American Psychiatric Press, 1987.

_____, Alexander C. McFarlane, and Lars Weisaeth, eds. *Traumatic Stress: The Effects of Overwhelming Experience on Mind, Body, and Society.* New York: Guilford Press, 1996.

van Dernoot, Peter. *Helping Your Children Cope with Your Cancer: A Guide for Parents and Families.* Long Island City, NY: Hatherleigh Press, 2002.

White, E.B. *Essays of E.B. White.* New York: Harper & Row, 1977.

ABOUT THE AUTHOR

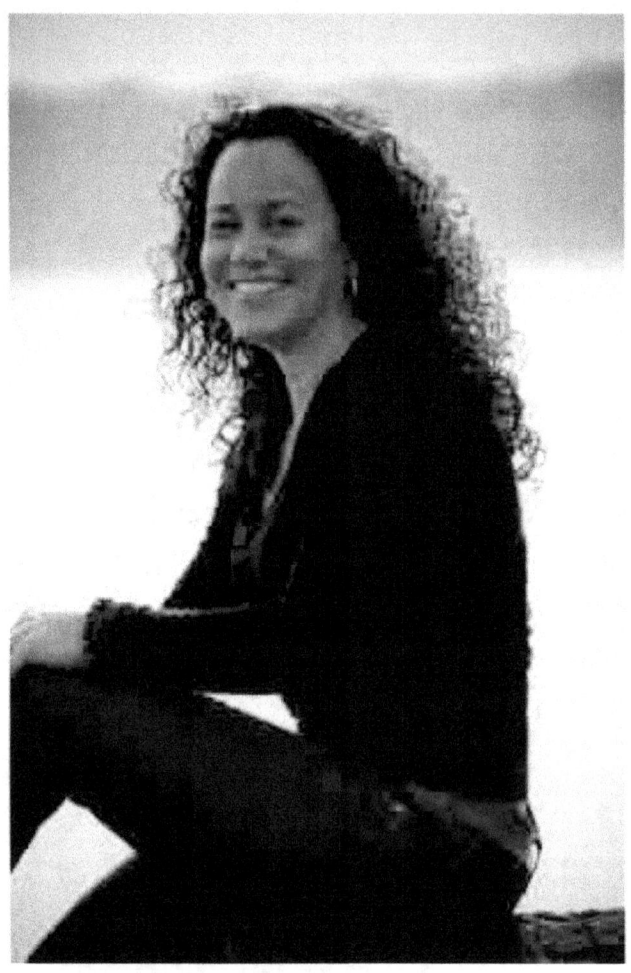

Figure II: Rebecca Douglas

Laura van Dernoot Lipsky has worked directly with trauma survivors for over two decades. At age 18, she regularly spent nights volunteering in a homeless shelter. From there, she went on to work with survivors of child abuse, domestic violence, acute trauma, and natural disasters. Simultaneously, she has been active in community organizing and movements for social and environmental justice and has taught on issues surrounding systematic oppression and liberation theory.

Like so many of her colleagues, Laura initially engaged in her work with great passion and commitment, and with a sense that it was a privilege to serve others. But over time, the worked changed her, until she was no longer the person she had once been. She felt a rising despair about the brutality of the world and anger at those who had helped to create the conditions of trauma and suffering of humans, animals, and our planet. About 10 years ago, she finally faced an uncomfortable reality: The work she cared so much about was taking a toll on her. Her work had compromised her ability to be present in her life, enjoy her relationships, and even be an effective social worker and educator.

Feeling that she could no longer work with integrity, she began the second stage of her involvement with trauma. In 2000, she quit her job as an emergency room social worker at Harborview Hospital in Seattle, Washington, and began an urgent quest for wisdom that would allow her to preserve her trust in life and its beauty even when doing work that guaranteed exposure to endless waves of pain. Her explorations took her from Buddhist monks and nuns to qigong healers to Native American medicine men and women to the latest scientific research on the effects of prolonged exposure to others' trauma. Laura's hunger to embrace both the joy and the sorrow of our life experiences is at the root of her concept of *trauma stewardship.*

Laura offered her first version of a workshop on trauma stewardship to a group of public health workers in 1999. Since then, she has trained a wide variety of people, including zookeepers and reconstruction workers in post-Katrina New Orleans, community organizers and health care providers in Japan, U.S. Air Force pilots, Canadian firefighters, public school teachers, and private practice doctors. She has worked locally, nationally, and internationally.

Recently, Laura turned her attention to the effects of trauma exposure on those doing frontline work in environmental and conservation movements throughout the world. She was among the first to talk publicly about the profound price that the witnessing of mass extinctions and other potentially irreversible ecological losses caused by global warming and other forms of human encroachment is exacting from the organizations and individuals who are attempting to save our planet.

In addition to traveling near and far as part of her dedication to support others in practicing trauma stewardship, Laura continues to consult with organizations and institutions while also maintaining a counseling practice. She volunteers in the public schools and is the founder and director of Prescolar Alice Francis, a Spanish-language preschool that is guided by a curriculum in social and environmental justice. Conducted entirely in Spanish, it is the only one of its kind in the Pacific

Northwest. Laura lives in Seattle, Washington, with her family; holds a master of social work degree; is bilingual in Spanish; and in 2008 was given a Yo! Mama award in recognition of her work as a community-activist mother. You can learn more about Laura and *Trauma Stewardship* at traumastewardship.com.

ABOUT BERRETT-KOEHLER PUBLISHERS

Berrett-Koehler is an independent publisher dedicated to an ambitious mission: Creating a World That Works for All.

We believe that to truly create a better world, action is needed at all levels—individual, organizational, and societal. At the individual level, our publications help people align their lives with their values and with their aspirations for a better world. At the organizational level, our publications promote progressive leadership and management practices, socially responsible approaches to business, and humane and effective organizations. At the societal level, our publications advance social and economic justice, shared prosperity, sustainability, and new solutions to national and global issues.

A major theme of our publications is "Opening Up New Space." They challenge conventional thinking, introduce new ideas, and foster positive change. Their common quest is changing the underlying beliefs, mindsets, and structures that keep generating the same cycles of problems, no matter who our leaders are or what improvement programs we adopt.

We strive to practice what we preach—to operate our publishing company in line with the ideas in our books. At the core of our approach is *stewardship,* which we define as a deep sense of responsibility to administer the company for the benefit of all of our "stakeholder" groups: authors, customers, employees, investors, service providers, and the communities and environment around us.

We are grateful to the thousands of readers, authors, and other friends of the company who consider themselves to be part of the "BK Community." We hope that you, too, will join us in our mission.

A BK Life Book

This book is part of our BK Life series. BK Life books change people's lives. They help individuals improve their lives in ways that are beneficial for the families, organizations, communities, nations, and world in which they live and work. To find out more, visit www.bk-life.com.

BE CONNECTED

Visit Our Website

Go to www.bkconnection.com to read exclusive previews and excerpts of new books, find detailed information on all Berrett-Koehler titles and authors, browse subject-area libraries of books, and get special discounts.

Subscribe to Our Free E-Newsletter

Be the first to hear about new publications, special discount offers, exclusive articles, news about bestsellers, and more! Get on the list for our free e-newsletter by going to www.bkconnection.com.

Get Quantity Discounts

Berrett-Koehler books are available at quantity discounts for orders of ten or more copies. Please call us toll-free at **(800) 929-2929** or email us at bkp.orders@aidcvt.com.

Host a Reading Group

For tips on how to form and carry on a book reading group in your workplace or community, see our website at www.bkconnection.com.

Join the BK Community

Thousands of readers of our books have become part of the "BK Community" by participating in events featuring our authors, reviewing draft manuscripts of forthcoming books, spreading the word about their favorite books, and supporting our publishing program in other ways. If you would like to join the BK Community, please contact us at bkcommunity@bkpub.com.

THE FIVE DIRECTIONS

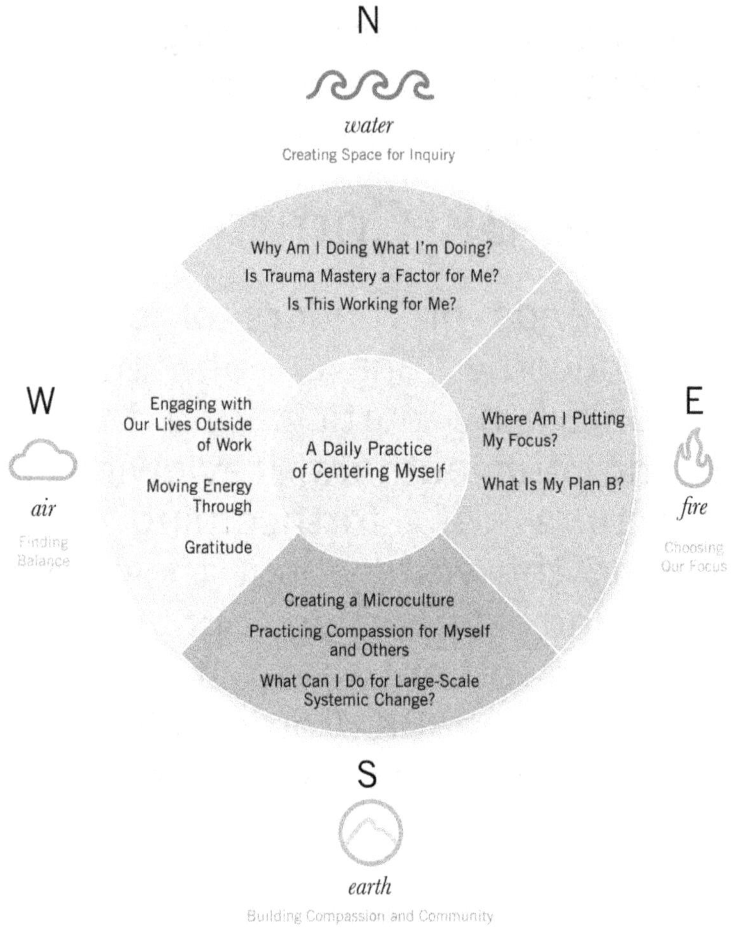

N

water
Creating Space for Inquiry

Why Am I Doing What I'm Doing?
Is Trauma Mastery a Factor for Me?
Is This Working for Me?

W

air
Finding Balance

Engaging with
Our Lives Outside
of Work

Moving Energy
Through
Gratitude

A Daily Practice
of Centering Myself

Where Am I Putting
My Focus?

What Is My Plan B?

E

fire
Choosing Our Focus

Creating a Microculture
Practicing Compassion for Myself and Others
What Can I Do for Large-Scale Systemic Change?

S

earth
Building Compassion and Community

Figure III

Index

A

accountability, lack of, *31*
activities,
 mindfulness while doing, *419, 421*
 for trauma mastery, *294*
addictions, *198, 200, 202, 204, 465*
Administration for Children's Services (ACS), *106*
adrenaline, *194, 200, 256*
advocacy, effectiveness of, *23*
Alice's Adventures in Wonderland (Carroll), *116*
alienation, *319*
alone time, *311*
Alvarado, Jorge, *274, 315*
Andersen, Heather, *422, 424, 427, 429*

Andersen Humor Model, *429*
anger or cynicism, *184, 186, 188, 190*
Animals Asia, *386*
animals' responses to threats, *409, 411*
animal welfare workers, *78, 79, 83, 86, 89, 90, 93, 95, 97, 106, 108, 136, 142, 145, 182, 194, 204, 206, 245, 299, 386, 434*
An Inconvenient Truth (Gore), *319*
answering to yourself, *155, 158*
antiviolence movement, *128, 132, 133, 135*
 See also domestic violence,
appreciation, *209*
Architecture for Humanity, *386, 388*
atrocities, *416*

attachments, *200*
attorneys, *98, 196, 334, 337, 340, 397*
Audubon Nature Institute, *136*
authenticity, *179*
awareness,
  cultivating, *70*
  living with, *416*
  self-, *245, 247, 331, 341*
  of trauma exposure response, *290*

B

balance,
  finding, *224, 409, 411, 414, 416, 419, 421*
  neutralizing imbalance, *174*
  returning to, *331*
  striving for, *409*
  through gratitude, *431*
bartering systems, *256*
Beardsley, Bill, *460*
bearing witness, *10, 414*

behavior,
  changes over time of, *33, 35*
  evaluating, *315, 317, 319, 321, 324*
  instinctive, *213*
  reasons for, *274, 276, 278*
  unethical, *31*
beliefs, unconscious, *447, 449*
bell time, *449, 452*
Benton, Dina, *194, 294*
binary structures, *124*
bisexual women, domestic violence among, *133*
Black Bear, Tillie, *133*
Boesak, Allan Aubrey, *38*
Book of Secrets, The (Chopra), *447*
boundaries, *20, 23*
Boyland, Deadria, *227, 230, 233, 235, 238, 240*
Bradford, Anna, *358, 360, 363, 365, 367, 370, 372*

breathing, deep, *419,*
421, 441
Bride, Brian, *63*
Brookins, John, *276,*
321
Brown, Margie, *429*
Brown, Warren, *151,*
153, 155, 158, 161
Buddhism, *218, 380, 382,*
435
Burk, Connie, *122,*
345, 348, 384
burnout, *238, 397*
Bush, George H.W.,
124, 126
Bush, George W.,
319

C

CakeLove, *151, 153, 155,*
158, 161
care, self-, *176, 221,*
224, 226, 367
caregivers,
  guilt feelings of, *68*
  self-care by, *224*
  stress of, *42*
Carroll, Lewis, *116*

Carter, Rubin
'Hurricane', *296, 328*
Casimire, R. Omar,
164
centering acts, *249,*
251
centering ourselves,
235, 238, 240, 241, 243, 245,
247, 249, 251, 253, 256, 258,
261, 263, 265, 267, 269, 271,
274, 276, 278, 281, 283, 285,
287, 290, 292, 294, 296, 299,
301, 302, 305, 307, 309, 311,
314, 315, 317, 319, 321, 324,
325, 327, 328, 331, 333, 334,
337, 340, 341, 344, 345, 348,
350, 352, 354, 356, 358, 360,
363, 365, 367, 370, 372, 374,
376, 378, 380, 382, 384, 386,
388, 390, 393, 395, 397, 400,
402, 404, 406, 408, 409, 411,
414, 416, 419, 421, 422, 424,
427, 429, 431, 434, 435, 438,
440, 441, 443, 445, 447, 449,
452, 473
change,
  awakening to, *6*
  fear of lack of, *82*

how to facilitate, *382, 384*
process of, *226*
resistance to, *116*
responsibility for, *384, 386*
systemic, *382, 384, 386, 388*
Chan Khong, *253*
chaos, *116*
child protective services (CPS) workers, *44, 186, 400, 453, 456, 458, 460, 463, 465, 467, 470, 472*
Chinese teachings, *245, 247, 409*
Chödrön, Pema, *213, 376*
Chopra, Deepak, *327, 447*
Cicero, *116*
Circles, *354, 467*
cognitive shifts, redefining your job, *26*
Cohen, Kenneth, *247*
collectives, *393*
commitment,
to jobs, *150*
to repairing the world, *400*
to self-care, *445*
without condition, *158*
to the work, *465, 467*
community,
bearing witness within, *414*
building, *224, 350, 352, 354, 356, 358*
compassion for self and others in, *374, 376, 378, 380*
microcultures, *350, 352, 354, 356, 358*
roles of our, *352, 354*
sharing loss with, *358, 360, 363*
systemic change, *382, 384, 386, 388*
systemic change through, *382*
compartmentalizing, *49*
compassion,
building, *350, 352, 354, 356, 358*

deepening our, *182, 184*
nature of, *382*
for ourselves and others, *6, 8, 299*
for self and others, *374, 376, 378, 380*
Compelled to Crime (Richie), *133*
competition, *141*
complexity, *120, 122, 124, 126, 128, 132, 133, 135*
conflicting feelings, *196, 198*
connections,
  with people you've helped, *356*
  personal, *23, 166, 168*
  to pets, *404, 406*
  undermining, *174*
consciousness levels, *247*
conscious oversight, *350, 352*
Conte, Jon, *190*
control,
  lack of, *292*
  need for, *440, 441*
  sense of personal, *221*
coping
  mechanisms, *224*
    See also defense mechanisms,
  defenses, *66, 68*
  dysfunctional, *256*
  expecting different outcomes, *292*
  minimizing, *136, 139, 141*
creativity,
  diminished, *114, 116, 118*
criminal justice workers, *253, 256, 258, 261, 263, 265*
crisis intervention workers, *164, 172*
crisis mode, *287*
criticism, self-, *317*
cultural issues,
  ancient traditions, *251*
  attitude toward jobs, *209*

creating negative culture, *139, 141*
culture of community as support, *354*
culture of gratitude, *434*
organizational culture, *28, 31, 139, 141, 209, 224, 305*
cumulative effects of trauma exposure, *35, 218*

D

Dalai Lama, *376*
Dance of Change, The (Senge), *350*
Dane County Time Bank, *256*
daVinci, Leonardo, *406*
debriefing, *233, 235, 305*
deep breathing, *419, 421, 441*
defense mechanisms, See also coping mechanisms;
warning signs of trauma exposure response, consequences of, *44*
denial, *68, 182, 370, 395*
disconnection, *182, 460*
dissociation, *59, 164, 166, 168*
intellectualization, *243, 245*
defensiveness, *465*
denial, *68, 182, 370, 395*
depression, *79*
despair, *97*
developing a Plan B, *341, 344, 345, 348*
deVries, Marten W., *354*
Dick, Rollie, *341*
diminished creativity, *114, 116, 118*
disconnection, *182, 460*
dis-ease, *409*
dissatisfaction, *106*
dissociation, *59, 164, 166, 168*

distancing from feelings, *70, 72*
doctors, *24*
domestic violence, criminalization of, *128, 132, 133, 135*
experiences of workers, *31, 108, 110, 122, 128, 132, 133, 135, 176, 227, 230, 233, 235, 238, 240, 253, 256, 258, 261, 263, 265, 400, 402*
doom, sense of, *86*
Douglas, Scott, *196*
Douglass, Frederick, *348*
dreams, sharing your, *344*
drug use, *194, 198, 200, 202, 204*
Dune, *180*

E

east or choosing focus, *224*
  consciousness of, *325, 327, 328, 331, 333*
  developing a Plan B, *341, 344, 345, 348*
  narrow focus, *82*
  shifting perspective for changing, *8, 10, 12*
efficacy, self-, *172*
Emerson, Ralph Waldo, *4*
emotional connections, *89, 204*
emotional health, *122*
emotions, allowing yourself to feel, *460, 463*
empathy, *20, 23, 76, 78, 79, 82, 136, 190, 192, 194, 196, 198, 243, 378*
empowerment, lack of, *79*
energy, *147, 409, 411, 414, 416, 419, 421*
enough-ness, *103, 106*
Environmental Home Center, *331, 333*
equanimity, *202*
exhaustion or physical problems, *142, 145, 147, 150*

experiences, reframing, *328*

F

Fadiman, Clifton, *424*
failure, *456*
faith, *226, 440, 441, 443*
family support, *311*
Farmer, Paul, *41*
fear, *180, 182, 184*
felt sense, *243*
feminism, *319*
firefighters, *44*
First Nations tribe, *352, 354*
first responders, *112*
Five Directions, *267, 269, 271*
Flateau, James B., *33*
focus,
  choosing, *224*
  consciousness of, *325, 327, 328, 331, 333*
  having too narrow, *82*
  shifting perspective for changing, *8, 10, 12*

Forest, James, *452*
Frank, Anne, *8*
Frankl, Viktor, *321, 324, 344*
freedom to change, *344*
free will, *341*
funerals, *358, 414, 424*

G

Gandhi, Mohandas K., *12*
Gangi, Robert, *33*
Garber, Judy, *79, 82*
Garvey, Marcus, *213*
Generon, *302, 305*
Gore, Al, *319*
grandiosity, *204, 206, 209*
gratitude, *431, 434, 435, 438*
greatness, *155*
Guevara, Che, *434*
guilt feelings,
  caregivers', *68*
  dealing with, *172, 174, 176, 179*
  effects of, *174*

work-related, *406, 408*
Gurganus, Alan, *434*
Gutiérrez, Gustavo, *38*

H
Hafiz, *180*
Halfkenny, Polly, *390, 393, 395, 397*
happiness, shame for feeling, *12*
Harborview Medical Center, *164*
hardship, approaches to, *331, 333*
Hartfield, Charlann, *350*
Hassan, Zaid, *302, 305, 307, 309, 311, 314, 321*
hate crimes, *108*
health, *305*
help, asking for, *393*
helping professions, *296*
helpless feelings, *10, 76, 78, 79, 82, 283*
Herman, Judith, *416*

heroic mode, *63*
Holocaust survivors, *172, 344*
homeostasis, *331*
honesty, *317*
honoring life, *226*
hooks, bell, *376*
hopeless feelings, *56, 76, 78, 79, 82*
Howell, Helen, *334, 337, 340*
Howell, Lem, *334*
H Street Skateboards, *345*
humility, *292, 431*
humor, *190, 422, 424, 427, 429*
Hurricane Katrina, *136, 294, 419*
hyperintellectualism, *243, 245*
hypervigilance, *108, 110, 112, 114, 440, 441*

I
idealism, *79, 145, 147*
ideal society, *41, 42*
identity, work as, *204, 206, 209*

imbalance, neutralizing, *174*
immigrant rights workers, *281, 283, 285, 287*
immunity from trauma exposure response, *63*
improvement, choosing, *8*
inadequacy, *98, 100, 103, 106, 108, 145*
Inconvenient Truth, An (Gore), *319*
indicators of trauma exposure response, *70*
inertia, *172*
inner well-being, *402*
Inova Regional Trauma Center, *354, 356*
inquiry,
    creating space for, *224, 274, 276*
    self-, *213, 215, 218, 220*
    space for, *315, 317, 319, 321, 324*
instinctive behaviors, *213*
intellectualization, *243, 245*
intention, creating, *447*
internal disarmament, *376*
internalized oppression, *100*
isolating yourself, *155, 168, 215, 218, 465*

J

James, William, *331*
Jansen, Golie, *23*
Jewish Federation, *108*
jobs,
    See also organizational culture,
    addiction to, *465*
    commitment to, *150*
    cultural issues of, *28, 31, 139, 141, 209*
    finding a calling, *321, 324*

finding passion for, *153, 155, 158, 161*
guilt at leaving, *179*
motivation for embracing, *317, 319, 356, 363, 365*
overwork, *200, 202*
service rationing, *24*
understanding effects of, *63*
us-versus-them mentality, *258*
wanting to stop, *319*
workplace dynamics, *120, 122*
Jung, Carl, *311*

K
Kabat-Zinn, Jon, *4*
Katrina, Hurricane, *136, 294, 419*
King, Martin Luther, Jr., *226*
Kingston, Maxine Hong, *122*
Knuth, Marianne, *386*
Kornfield, Jack, *218, 331, 374, 414*
Kufunda, *386*

L
Lan, Luo, *106, 108*
laughter, *429*
law enforcement personnel, *147, 150*
Lawson, Billie, *120, 122, 218, 419*
lawyers, *98, 196, 334, 337, 340, 397*
learned helplessness, *172*
Learning as Leadership, *470*
Leitch, Laurie, *63*
LeRoy, Andree, *42*
lesbians, domestic violence among, *133*
Levine, Peter, *68, 213, 243, 409, 411*
Levine, Stephanie, *112, 114*
Lewen, Donna, *281, 283, 285, 287*
liberation theory, *38, 41*

life outside work, *400, 402, 404, 406, 408*
lifestyle, *221*
Lips, Karen, *76*
Lipsky, Michael, *24, 26*
listening, *162*
Liu Dong, *245, 247, 251*
Loeffler, Kati, *142, 145*
loving-kindness meditation, *376, 378*

M

Malcolm, *356*
Man's Search for Meaning (Frankl), *321, 324*
Maples, Cheri, *253, 256, 258, 261, 263, 265*
Marsalis, Branford, *70*
Martin, Lesra, *328*
martyrdom, *14, 147*
mastery of trauma, *292, 294, 296, 299, 301, 365, 431*
McFarlane, Alexander C., *42, 44*
meaningful tasks, *221*

meditations, *376, 378, 419, 421*
Merton, Thomas, *198*
microcultures, *350, 352, 354, 356, 358*
military personnel, *186*
Miller-Karas, Elaine, *110*
mindfulness,
  definitions, *4*
  doing activities with, *419, 421*
  reasons for behavior, *274, 276, 278*
mindfulness bells, *449, 452*
minimizing feelings or events, *136, 139, 141, 174*
mistreatment, *168*
Mooney, James, *168, 315*
Mooney, Linda, *294*
Moore, Jonathan, *285, 287*
motivation, *274, 296, 302*

N

Native American Ceremonies, *315*
Native Americans, First Nations Tribe, *352, 354*
 spirituality of, *294*
 traditions of, *267, 269, 416, 467*
 violence among, *133*
natural disasters, *136, 294, 419*
nature solos, *305*
negativism, *139, 141, 327*
Newcomb, Charles, *245*
Newsweek, *166*
NewYork Times Magazine, *31*
Nhat Hanh, Thich, *124, 126, 176, 218, 253, 256, 258, 416, 435*
NiCarthy, Ginny, *206*
Niebuhr, Reinhold, *434*
Nietzsche, Friedrich, *274*
No Child Left Behind Act, *24*
north or space for, inquiry, *224*
 evaluating behavior, *315, 317, 319, 321, 324*
 mastery of trauma, *292, 294, 296, 299, 301*
 mindfulness of reasons for behavior, *274, 276, 278*
Northwest Immigrant Rights Project (NWIRP), *281, 283, 285, 287, 290*
Northwest Network of Bisexual, Trans, Lesbian and Gay Survivors of Abuse, *116, 118*
not enoughness, *98, 100, 103, 106, 108*

O

obligations, *145*
obstacles, seeing paths around, *168, 172*

opening inquiry, *213, 215, 218, 220*
oppression,
  forms of, *100, 103*
  role in trauma of, *38*
  systematic, *38, 41, 44, 186*
oppressive messages, *98, 100*
organizational culture, *28, 31, 139, 141, 209, 224, 305*
organizations,
  covert emotional life of, *467*
  cultures of, *139, 141, 209, 224*
  roles in trauma stewardship of, *23, 24, 26, 28, 31, 33, 35*
overwhelming feelings, *82, 142, 164, 172, 456*
overwork, *200, 202*

P

Pantesco, Victor, *76*
paradoxes, *10, 26*
paramedics, *46*
Parry, Cindy, *46, 49, 51, 54, 56, 59*
passion, finding, *153, 155, 158, 161*
patience, *226*
People of Color Against AIDS Network, *28, 31*
People's Hurricane Relief Fund, *419*
People's Institute for Survival and Beyond, *419*
persecution, *168, 172*
personal control, *221*
personal dynamics, *19, 20, 23*
personal history, *302*
personal life, *164, 200, 202*
Petersen, John, *182*
Plan B, *341, 344, 345, 348*
policies, effective, *28*
pollution metaphor, *35, 38*

posttraumatic stress disorder (PTSD), *63, 224*
power, abusing, *35*
powerlessness, *89*
practice, steps toward, *447, 449, 452, 453*
presence in the experience,
  bell-ringing tradition for, *449*
  cultivating quality of, *211, 213*
  for healing process, *70*
  mindfulness for, *4*
  nonantagonistic, *168, 172*
  openness to, *176, 179*
practice of, *251*
primary trauma, *296, 302*
prison inmates, *132, 256, 258, 296*
prison workers, *33, 276*
Proust, Marcel, *325*

Psychological Trauma (van der Kolk), *221*
public health workers, *172*
public views of trauma responders, *42, 44*

Q
qigong, *245, 247, 374, 419*

R
rape laws, *128, 132*
reactions, habitual, *311*
reality, perceptions of, *452*
Rebuild, *354, 356*
reflection, self-, *249*
reframing experiences, *328, 414, 416*
relationships,
  emotional presence in, *108*
  for trauma mastery, *294*
relaxation, *406*
relief, lack of, *82*

resiliency, *460, 463*
resolutions for happiness, *155, 158*
resourcing, *328, 331*
responsibility, *82, 309*
Rice, A.K., *467*
Richards, Kimberley, *419*
Richie, Beth E., *31, 133*
Robinson, Jill, *386*
roles, negotiating, *120, 122*
Roshi, Suzuki, *6*
Rosten, Leo, *427*
Roy, Arundhati, *386*
Rumi, *344*
rumination, *354*
Rwandan genocide, *10*

S

sainthood, *434*
Sanders, Kerry, *31, 33*
sangha, *350*
scarcity, *100, 103*
Schwartz, Karyn, *206, 209*
Schwegel, Bob, *166*
scientists, *95, 245*
Sealth, Chief, *378*
secondary posttraumatic stress disorder (PTSD), *63*
self-awareness, *245, 247, 331*
self-care, *176, 221, 224, 226, 367*
self-efficacy, *172*
self-inquiry, *213, 215, 218, 220*
self-reflection, *249*
self-transformation process, *4*
Seligman, Martin E.P., *79, 82*
Senge, Peter, *350, 352*
sense of humor, *424*
service rationing, *24, 26*
service to others, *321, 324*
shamanic traditions, *352*
Shantideva, *200*

sharing trauma, *372,
414, 460, 463*
Shiva, Vandana, *38*
Siegel, Daniel, *4, 245,
331*
Sinclair, Cameron,
386, 388
sleep, *247, 249, 408*
slowing down, *416*
social norms, *186*
social support, *221*
societal impacts on trauma
stewardship, *35, 38, 41,
42, 44*
somatic experiencing, *328, 331,
411*
south or building compassion and community, *224*
   microcultures, *350,
   352, 354, 356, 358*
   practicing compassion for self and others,
   374, 376, 378, 380
   systemic change,
   382, 384, 386, 388

Spence, Harry, *453,
456, 458, 460, 463, 465, 467,
470, 472*
spirituality, *267*
Stade, Kirsten, *78*
Star Wars: Episode I—The Phantom Menace, *180, 182*
Stifter, Vicky, *281,
283, 285, 287*
stillness, finding,
249, 251
Stohr, Kate, *386, 388*
Street-Level Bureaucracy (Lipsky), *24*
street-level bureaucrats, *26, 28*
stress, resistance to, *221, 224*
structural violence,
38, 41
Suarez, Ray, *66*
success, envisioning, *155*
suffering, *14, 16, 376*
Sufi wisdom, *376*
suicide, *26, 440*

Sultanoff, Steven, *424, 429*
support,
  from community, *352, 354, 356*
  culture of, *224*
  family, *311*
  need for, *309, 311*
  social, *221*
  for trauma exposure response, *28*
  from your organization, *23*
systematic oppression, *38, 41, 44, 186*
systemic change, *382, 384, 386, 388*

T

traditions of, *241, 243*
taking sides, *120, 122, 141*
Taoism, *245*
Tatum, Diane, *176*
Tavistock Institute, *467*

Taylor-Murphy, Kanika, *419*
teachers, *24, 28*
teamwork models, *458*
Ternasky, Mike, *345*
Thanassi, Mark, *411*
threat responses, *409, 411, 424*
Through the Looking Glass (Carroll), *116*
Thurber, James, *429*
tikkun olam, *388*
Tomlin, Lily, *190*
transformation, *See* change, transformation,
self-, *4*
trauma,
  acknowledging exposure to, *68, 70*
  being the creator of, *456*
  effects of, *14, 227, 230*
  first-hand experience with, *296, 302*

mastery of, *292, 294, 296, 299, 301, 431*
Trauma Center (Boston, Massachusetts), *147, 150*
trauma exposure response,
  definition, *62*
  identification with, *76*
  keeping positive, *72*
  methods for dealing with, *230*
  occurrences of, *63*
Trauma First Aide, *110, 112*
Traumatic Stress (deVries), *354*
Traumatic Stress (van der Kolk and McFarlane), *44*
trust, *441*
Truth and Reconciliation Commission, *66*
Tum, Rigoberta Menchú, *38*
Tutu, Desmond, *66, 384, 467*

U
unconscious beliefs, *447, 449*
unethical behavior, *31*
U.S. Air Force personnel, *186*
  See also military personnel,
U.S. Department of Health and Human Services, *151*
U.S. Department of Justice (DOJ), *132*

V
van der Kolk, Bessel A., *42, 44, 221, 224, 296, 467*
veterinarians, *142, 145, 245*
violence, structural, *38, 41*
violence prevention workers, *112, 116, 118*
Vitaliano, Peter, *42*

Vredenburg, Vance, *83, 86, 89, 90, 93, 95, 97*
vulnerability, *182, 460*

W
Wake, David, *90*
Waking the Tiger (Levine), *68, 411*
warning signs of trauma exposure response,
  addictions, *198, 200, 202, 204*
  anger or cynicism, *184, 186, 188, 190*
  avoidance, *78, 162, 164, 435*
  diminished creativity, *114, 116, 118*
  dissociation, *59, 164, 166, 168*
  dissociative moments, *164, 166, 168*
  exhaustion or physical problems, *142, 145, 147, 150*
  fear, *180, 182, 184*
  grandiosity, *204, 206, 209*
  guilty feelings, *172, 174, 176, 179*
  hypervigilance, *108, 110, 112, 114*
  inability to embrace complexity, *120, 122, 124, 126, 128, 132, 133, 135*
  inadequacy, *98, 100, 103, 106, 108*
  minimizing feelings or events, *136, 139, 141*
  sense of persecution, *168, 172*
wave metaphor, *325, 327*
Way of Qigong, The (Cohen), *247*
wellness path, *402, 404, 411*
west or finding,

balance, *224*
energy, *409, 411, 414, 416, 419, 421*
gratitude, *431, 434, 435, 438*
life outside work, *400, 402, 404, 406, 408*
Wilson, Ed, *247*
Wisconsin Coalition Against Domestic Violence, *253*
Wonder, Stevie, *16*
worldview, *63, 317, 327*

X
X, Malcolm, *16*

Y
Yawnghwe, Harn, *182, 184*
yuan shen, *245, 247*

www.ingramcontent.com/pod-product-compliance
Lightning Source LLC
Chambersburg PA
CBHW071011180325
23651CB00071B/975